REFLECTING ON THERAPY

REFLECTING ON THERAPY

Michael Jacobs

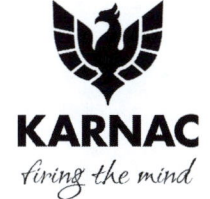

KARNAC
firing the mind

First published in 2024 by
Karnac Books Limited
62 Bucknell Road
Bicester
Oxfordshire OX26 2DS

British Library Cataloguing in Publication Data

A C.I.P. for this book is available from the British Library

978-1-80013-271-9 (paperback)
978-1-80013-272-6 (e-book)
978-1-80013-273-3 (PDF)

Typeset by Medlar Publishing Solutions Pvt Ltd, India

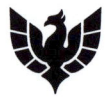

www.firingthemind.com

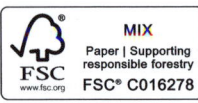

Turn the page for the first reflection.

Space is left for the reader who wishes to add their own thoughts to mine.

1

There's no hurry—how you might use these reflections

Counselling (or psychotherapy) is not a miracle cure, although you might think so, the way some people throw the concept around as the solution to all mental problems. It is a slow process. Bar a miracle or a disaster we change slowly and need time to develop. One session, one week at a time. There must be time to reflect between sessions, both by the client and the therapist. There is so much pressure these days to get through the waiting list, or to deal with a crippling issue in a short-term contract: six weeks to change someone's habits or the anxieties of a lifetime?

I just ask: could we all slow down?

That's the way I suggest you use this book: slowly, one page at a time, naturally. But more than that: one reflection a week perhaps. Give yourself time to ponder, to add your own thoughts if you wish. If there is anything in what I write, it is best to savour it, to develop it, or disagree with it. To reflect rather than look to this book for answers.

Taking it one step at a time applies to the practice of therapy too. There may be a feeling that you ought to be able to process everything your client tells you over the course of a single session. Or that you should address everything the client tells you within the therapeutic hour. If you can get hold of one thing in the hour, that's great. If your client can, that's even greater. You may be a genius and understand everything the client is saying, but your client is probably finding it difficult enough dealing with one issue each week, even though your client is telling you about all the others as well.

If you can get hold of something that rings a bell, that looks like it's important in understanding the client, then hold it in mind, let it enter your imagination and memory as you watch and listen. Allow yourself to play with it, in the session if you can, but if not, in quiet moments in the week; and see what else comes to mind. You may be taking the wrong road, but it is sometimes the road you haven't ventured down before that leads to a good place. Yet slowly does it, let it settle, wonder what it is that you have caught on to. And if it seems right, and at the right time, offer it to your client. Depending on how your client responds, pursue it together.

So, stop reading here, put the book down. If you wish, you can read this reflection again; but wait until some other time, perhaps as much as a week, to turn to the next.

Slow down …

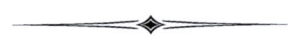

Your thoughts

2

'How are you?'

Many clients care about their therapists. So when they ask 'How are you?' at the start of their session this is not just a pleasantry, nor is it necessarily a way of breaking the ice—though there can be that to it too. They want to know if their therapist is all right, alive enough, alert enough, and free enough of their own concerns, to be able to attend to them. I once made the mistake of thinking that it was essential for me to be present for an unhappy client, despite my having the most dreadful cold. So I dragged myself into work. Within a minute the client realised that I was not well, and she said quite forcibly she did not want to go on with the session, and that I should be back at home and look after myself. She was right, and I knew it really, because I had already decided I was going to cancel all the other sessions that particular day. Her need might have been great, but she also needed me to be well enough to contain what she would bring to the session.

I once had to spend a few weeks in hospital. When I resumed my practice one of my clients was particularly angry that I had not let her know when we would be resuming therapy. I had not known either. But it wasn't simply that she was angry with me for not being there for her. What was clear was that she was worried how I was faring during my absence. I should have let her know.

These are important moments, which support what Harold Searles says about the way patients can be therapists to their analyst.[1] Searles argues that the therapist needs to be able to accept the patient's unconscious therapeutic efforts towards the analyst. He even suggests that the client/therapist roles can be reversed, with the client observing aspects of the therapist's countertransference that need to be addressed if the therapist is to help the client.

It is not surprising therefore that 'How are you?' can be an indication of the need in the client to test the water, wondering perhaps without realising it (or in the case of my client, not even unconsciously) whether they need to go easy on the therapist, or whether the therapist is indeed well enough to fully accept what the client wants to unload. 'I want you to be well—I care how you are—because how

---

[1] Searles, H. (1999). The patient as therapist to his analyst. In: *Countertransference and Related Subjects: Selected Papers* (pp. 380–459). Madison, CT: International Universities Press.

you are makes all the difference as to whether you will be able to care for me in the way I need.'

I may be a wounded healer but my client wants to be sure I am well enough.

Your thoughts

3

Being outrageous

'Sometimes I find myself getting very bored.' 'It was the last session of the day and I was very tired.' 'I don't look forward to that particular client at all, since she is so bland.' Reports I have heard in supervision.

Blandness is quite infectious. As therapists we try to be alert and understanding, so it is disturbing to be dragged down into a narcotic state where we cease to give the client our full attention, and by and large sit out the session, glad that at least the client can talk, even if the story is quite devoid of any feeling. It can be like that week after week, client and therapist loyally committed to the time together, both aware that little is happening, and that nothing is apparently changing. Neither say anything about it, because the therapist does not want to offend the client and the client does not want to offend the therapist. Yes, the client feels it too, but is afraid, as in every other part of life, to make a fuss about it, and so obediently attends and talks;

and talks; and talks; and thinks that's what therapy is all about.

We might find the reason lies in the client having become compliant: 'Don't cause a fuss, just go along with it'. The therapist picks this up from the client and becomes compliant too, doing little or nothing to shake the client into something livelier and more interesting.

Shake the client? Surely not? But as I listen to my supervisee describing how the sessions go, that's one of the images that comes to my mind. I want to shake them. The client? Or the supervisee? Perhaps both. Of course, I do not mean to be taken literally: that would be outrageous. I even suppress the idea for a few moments, thinking I shouldn't say that to my supervisee. Am I also being dragged into the morass of ordinariness and caution? So I share the thought—not, of course, as advice, as to *what* to say, but to suggest that what my supervisee might try *to do* is first to shake themselves out of the fog of compliance, and be a little outrageous. A *little* outrageous, I stress. For example, what might the therapist say relatively easily to other clients, which would be outrageous to this client? 'I'm feeling pretty angry (sad, happy, amused) about that', and then adding, 'But you don't appear to feel anything at all'; or 'Is it unsafe with me to show me what you really feel?'

Or even: 'That's outrageous. Don't you feel that too?'

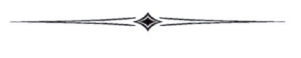

Your thoughts

4

Saying 'No'

It probably goes against the grain in someone whose profession involves helping others to have to say 'No'; and, we might add, saying 'No more'. Yet it is important both for our own well-being as well as for the good of the person to whom we are having (in the gentlest way, at least at first) to say 'No', or even 'No more'.

There are a number of situations where this is an essential response. The most obvious is when someone wants therapy, is willing to pay for it, and yet from the initial assessment appears to be completely unsuitable for what the therapist can offer. This may be because the presenting issues are so intractable that it is almost exploitative to offer what that particular therapist can provide, when it is ninety per cent obvious that it will not get anywhere near touching the underlying deep-seated issue. Of course there is always hope, that something will break through at some point, which miraculously shifts the situation for the client. But should therapists believe in miracles?

A somewhat more hopeful variant is that this particular therapist does not have the training, the experience, and the enthusiasm to work with specific presenting issues. There should be others who can, or who can at least assess more accurately whether what they offer would be a possible way forward. That is why a therapist would be wise to have knowledge of others in the profession who offer an alternative approach, and to whom referral might be made—not as a last resort, however, but as a positive and hopeful way forward for the client.

In turn that means recognising not just the strength of someone's cry for help, and how it can appeal to an innate wish to make things better for those in pain and difficulty. It also means acknowledging the power of the omnipotent fantasy: the belief that the efficacy of a chosen approach to therapy, or the conviction that I can take on anything, or both, can blind a therapist to their obvious deficiencies, which we all have. While it is true that every new client will teach us more about how to work, and that experience of new situations and new issues enlarges our knowledge and extends our skills, we also cannot use that excuse to justify the mistakes we will inevitably make which damage the client; or to exploit the client because we need the work.

It is difficult to resist the appeal of those who tug at our heartstrings, or who challenge us to take them on and prove what good therapists we think we are. Yet when there is any doubt about working with a particular issue or client, as good therapists this should strengthen the resolve to say 'No'.

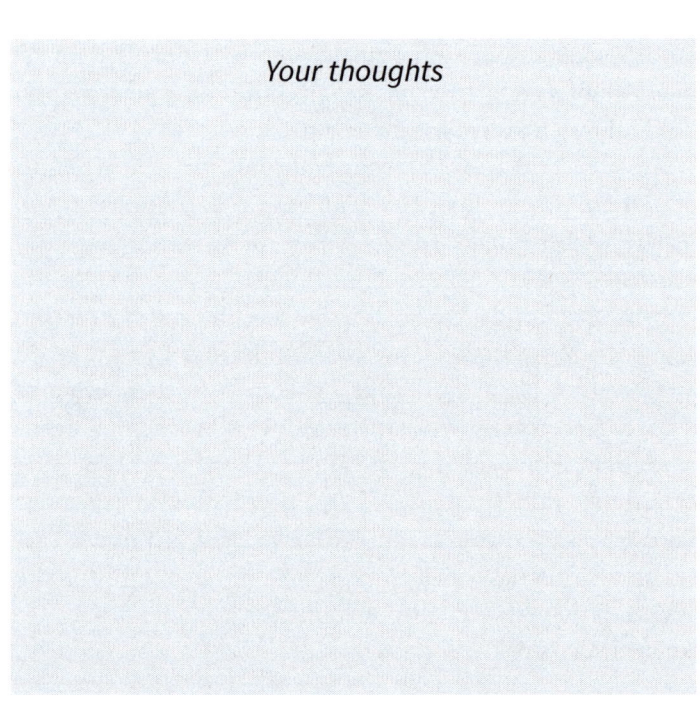

Your thoughts

5

Developing practice

In Lampedusa's novel *The Leopard*,[2] faced with the prospect of a revolution in Sicily, Count Falconeri says: 'If we want things to stay as they are, things will have to change.' For hundreds of years Sicily had been ruled by the Bourbons but was passing into new governance following Garibaldi's invasion.

It is a paradox, of course, for how can it all stay the same and still change? For myself it raises the question of what might need to change in my thinking and practice if I am going to go on being a useful practitioner. We might imagine that those who have recently completed their training will be *au fait* with all the latest thinking about practice and all the latest theories that inform our work, and therefore do not face change. Nevertheless, there is a

---

[2] Lampedusa, G. T. (2007). *The Leopard*, A. Colquhoun (Trans.). London: Vintage Classics.

question about how much those who have taught and supervised new therapists have been up to date themselves; and how much they have been willing to teach developments not just in their own school (where they themselves trained) but in other therapeutic schools. I wonder, as far as my own discipline is concerned, how much different psychodynamic trainings have recognised the huge changes that have taken place in psychoanalysis over the last forty years.

Most of us look back on our training as sacrosanct. It gave us clear guidance how to think and practice as we somewhat shakily encountered our first clients. It held us safe in the confusing world of human unhappiness. It was reassuring to have all that knowledge at our back. The longer our training (and it can extend for many years) the more we are likely to be wedded to it. It has, after all, cost us a lot of money and a lot of effort.

We may have chosen supervisors who would reinforce the learning we had received. We may have latched on to what seemed like certainties, forgetting that (in the best trainings) we had been encouraged to think broadly, and to ask questions of what we were taught. As our practice developed we may have added the odd skill here and there, but basically we remained the same. There is a certain tribalism about the world of therapy, and we feel more secure staying in our own tribe, not particularly interested in how other tribes think and work.

As we become more secure in our practice, do we become more fixed in our ideas of best practice and the most cogent theories? Or do we look, from that established position, at what is new and what we might change in our thinking and practice, if we are to remain the same?

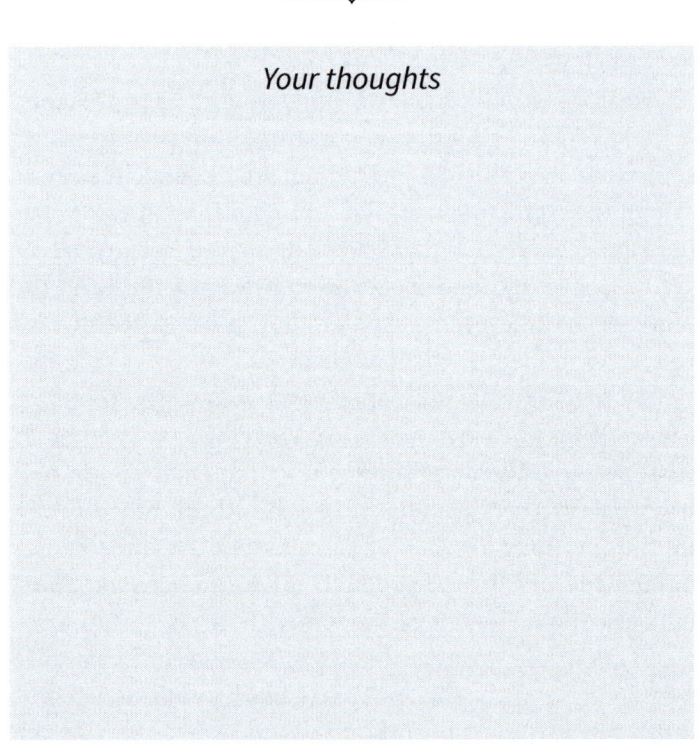

Your thoughts

6

Emptying and opening

There is a theological debate (bear with me!) around a Greek word 'kenosis'. It sort of means 'emptying', and features in discussions about how much Christ emptied himself (since he was thought to be divine) when he became human. It is relevant to our work as therapists, inasmuch as I wonder how much we need to empty ourselves in order to be more fully open to those who come for help.

This is not an unfamiliar notion in those who write about being a therapist. Remember how Carl Rogers is said to have opened a window at the end of each session and breathed in fresh air to prepare himself to see the next person. It is as if he needed to set aside (though I am sure not to forget) the person he had just seen in order to be open to the next. In the psychoanalytic tradition, Wilfred Bion wrote of the need for therapists to impose upon themselves 'a positive discipline of eschewing memory or desire'.[3] This doesn't just mean avoiding the temptation to impose an agenda on themselves or on the client. It also means being constantly open to hearing or sensing something new from the client. This may of course throw all that you have thought about a person into confusion, as you pick up something you have never considered relevant before.

What is particularly significant about Bion's wish to set aside memory or desire is that he looked beyond knowledge to a state of faith where we try to let go of knowledge. This ties in with that obscure theological discussion of how much Christ emptied himself of his divine knowledge to become human, an interesting parallel. All our training has emphasised knowledge: theories about people, and knowledge of appropriate skills. This we draw upon as we try to understand what the client is telling us—how it 'fits' with what we have learned; as well as how we should best respond, according to all that we have been trained to say or do.

What I am suggesting is that if we wish to be as open as possible to what a client is telling or showing us, we may want to consider those times when we have to empty ourselves of everything we have learned, because in the end

---

[3] Bion, W. R. (1970). *Attention and Interpretation*. London: Tavistock, p. 31.

what probably contributes most to the value of a therapist is that they are someone who has listened, and worked with many people; has been open to them, and has become soaked in so many dimensions of human experience; and (here is the paradox) that wealth of experience allows a therapist to be immersed in the engagement between two people, without conscious effort, without thinking what to say or do. But it needs faith in the client and ourselves to work that way.

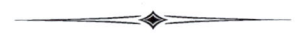

Your thoughts

7

What is expertise?

It seems to me that the emphasis on training and particularly on more and more post-qualification training, is that it suggests that therapists need to develop more and more expertise, and know more and more about the latest ideas and practices. As a result it is all too easy to forget that the real expert in the therapy room is the client! After all, clients come to therapy knowing what troubles them: they know how they feel, and what they are thinking, what hurts and what relieves them. They may be less sure that the solution to their issues lies within themselves. The task of the therapist is firstly to create a relationship where it becomes increasingly possible to talk openly to each other; and secondly to forge a working relationship where the therapist encourages the client to take the initiative, rather than perpetuating the client's initial expectation that it is the therapist who will make it all better.

It is not difficult to talk about passing the initiative to the client, although I suspect much more difficult to actually remember to do it. The client expects wisdom from the therapist; and everything that our training and post-qualification education tends to reinforce are our own expectations that we should know how to address every issue that arises. So what might we say and do that enables our clients to foster and develop their own expertise about themselves?

Firstly, listen for any hint that the client is looking themselves for an answer to their own experience. A little judicious questioning may help them to extend their descriptions of what they felt or are still feeling, what the circumstances were in which they had such and such experience: what it was like, what it might have reminded them of, etc. A further step is to invite the client to consider their own ideas about why they might have felt the way they did, what they thought, or what they said. It is of course right to avoid too many questions, and what I am thinking of here is a much quieter, tentative way of offering client the space and the support to think more widely, perhaps think out of the box, in the way that a teacher would want to encourage the learner to think something for themselves. Not an interrogation, but an invitation.

I stress that the invitation is to explore, to gently dig around, to engage in what used to be thought of as 'self-analysis', knowing that the therapist is there for support; and, as the client begins to take over this self-exploration, expertise shifts from therapist to client in a co-operative venture towards self-knowledge.

Your thoughts

29

8

Balancing the ship

Joseph Conrad, author and master mariner, writes in one of his memoirs, *The Mirror of the Sea*, of the need to load the cargo in sailing ships in such a way as to balance the ship, since there was no other ballast than the goods the ship was to carry. The chief mate needed to check that the ship settled in the water with neither fore nor aft too low or high, and neither listing to port or starboard. But every ship in his experience was slightly different, and the chief mate who got used to the ship would know to adjust the balance: a little more forward or aft, a little more to port or starboard; because when it came to sailing through rough seas and howling gales each ship behaved differently. If she was loaded well, she would ride the waves and brave the storm, stable because she was perfectly balanced when loaded in port.

It was that note about loading the cargo to balance the ship, and that all ships are different, that struck me as interesting. Is there such a person as a perfectly balanced individual? Of course not, but it might be one of the objectives of therapy: to take Conrad's image of the individually balanced ship and apply it to what balances us sufficiently to be able to cope with the storms that life inevitably brings. Each person reacts differently to those stresses: just as a balanced diet varies from person to person; just as the balance of work and leisure varies from person to person; and just as the ratio of activity to passivity will be different. And the right balance is perhaps only tested properly when there is a crisis, when we are thrown about, and when we look to achieve what stability we can.

It may be one of the aims of therapy to help clients work out for themselves how to find the right balance in the different aspects of their life, one that will help see them through the present crisis and the one that is yet to come. It is, however, something clients need to find for themselves, since each person is unique, and each person's set of circumstances is unique. It is also a task for a therapist, to find what is the right balance for themselves, in terms of the number of clients, the amount of time for others outside therapy, the best balance between studying people on the one hand and learning about things other than therapy on the other, the right balance between this very sedentary occupation and the need for a more active pursuit.

Your thoughts

9

And …?

It was a little tip that I picked up almost inadvertently from a colleague. It was a time when we were talking during a coffee break, and I was chatting away about my weekend. I was listing some of the things I had been able to get done, and I ended up with an 'and'. I can't remember precisely but it was something like: 'I managed to get the lawn cut, and we also had a walk, and …'

And I stopped, at which point my colleague said 'and?', and I realised that I had been about to tell her about someone I met, whom I knew she wasn't very keen on.

But that doesn't matter. The point is that I had stopped talking at that little word 'and', when clearly, when I uttered it, I had intended to say more. And very simply, and rather neatly, my colleague had invited me to complete what I was going to say. I can't remember now whether I actually went on to tell her about meeting the person she didn't like or not. What I do remember was how it struck me that by stopping at 'and', I was on that occasion censoring the next thing I wanted to say.

It was obvious to me that I was pretty consciously censoring my words. But I thought what a gentle and effective way my colleague had of encouraging me to finish my sentence. She did not know, of course, whether or not I had stopped myself talking about something difficult; whether or not I stopped because I thought I might be boring her; or whether or not I had deliberately or unconsciously censored what I had intended to say. She simply could see that there was something else, and very gently she gave me an opening to complete the sentence.

And how useful it was, just to repeat that one little word 'and', rather than saying 'go on', which would have felt in the circumstances rather more hectoring. It allowed me to choose either to finish what I had, in one way, wanted to say; or to check myself by saying 'It doesn't matter'.

So now I am more aware when someone is talking to me that if they stop with an 'and' (or a 'but', etc.), there may well be more that could be said; and that I can invite them to continue, if they wish, to tell me what they had thought of saying; also wondering, for my part, whether it was something they thought I might not want to hear.

Your thoughts

10

More than a parrot

Through his close observation of mothers and their babies (and it tended to be mothers), Daniel Stern observes the differences in the way parents can respond to their infants, somewhere around the age 9–15 months.[4] Parents invariably mirror what their infant child is expressing, but some do this rather mechanically, imitating sounds that the infant has made, or mirroring the infant's physical (mainly facial) expressions.

As straightforward feedback, this copying conveys little. It tells the infant that the parent has heard and has observed what the baby has expressed in various sounds and facially, but it does not convey to their child that the parent knows what the child is expressing because the parent has had a similar experience. As Stern writes:

---

[4] Stern, D. N. (1985). *The Interpersonal World of the Infant*. New York: Basic Books, pp. 138–142.

'Strict imitation alone won't do'. A much more helpful response needs the parent first of all to be able to 'read' the infant, and then to engage with the infant in a way that adds something to the 'conversation'; because it wouldn't be much of a conversation between two adults if we simply repeated word for word, and tone for tone, what the other person has said to us.

In the case of parent and child the parent adds something in their response which Stern calls 'affective attunement'. He gives several examples of this, but the one that stands out is the response of one mother who, as her little ten-month-old girl flings herself about joyfully, says forcefully, 'YES, thatta girl'. Not 'Yes, thatta girl', but 'YES, thatta girl'. It's the mother's enthusiastic response which is so marked.

I note the age when these interactions are so important: 9–15 months, when parents who are attuned to their babies pick up a way of responding that is different to the more imitative responses typical of the first few months of their interactions. This suggests that in our therapeutic conversations, adult to adult, it may in the first instance be enough to mirror the client, repeating words and phrases, summarising and paraphrasing; but that as we get more of a measure of the client, our responses need to be those which convey something of our own responses, so that we are more deliberately becoming attuned to what we are hearing and being told.

That doesn't mean responding with our own stories as we might in more ordinary conversations, but it does mean responding in such a way as to show that we have not just heard, not just understood, but have been actually able to share in the client's experience, expressing ourselves as well as reflecting back what the client has said.

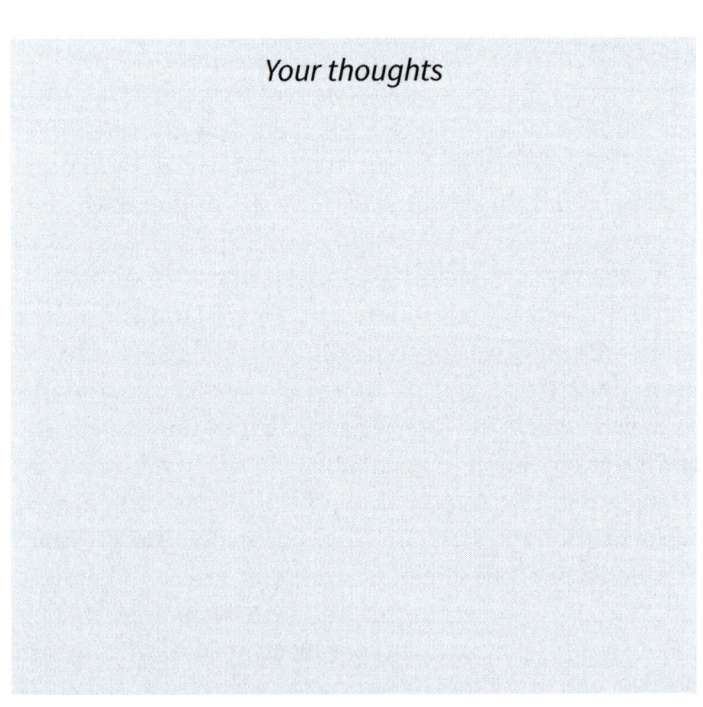

Your thoughts

11

Quick to judge

There was a man who for several years called himself Thomas Quick, during which time he confessed in his therapy sessions to a number of unsolved murders—thirty in all. He was seen as Sweden's most prolific serial killer. He seemed to know details about the cases which had apparently not been made public—or that was the way the detectives saw it. He identified the murder weapon wrongly in one case, but he went on guessing until he got it right.

He was tried and found guilty of eight murders. But after a while he stopped co-operating with the authorities, and changed his name back to the one he had grown up with. A documentary maker, examining all these cases, realised that there was not a scrap of evidence that proved he was responsible. Indeed, as they picked over his evidence, he had misidentified details about the victims. It transpired he had dug out information that was in public libraries, which made it look to his interrogators that he knew about them from personal experience.

There is so much that could be said about this. It was not false memory syndrome, because 'Quick' made it clear that he had made it all up in therapy in order to get more attention. He'd read about mental illness and realised that the more lurid patients' symptoms and stories, the more attention they got. It seems that he had up to then had a very lonely life.

The more I reflect upon even these brief details of what became known as the Thomas Quick Affair, the more I think how much this tells us as therapists. Is it that there are really interesting clients, whose stories grab our attention; which I am not denying are probably true—but are they sometimes embellished? And are there people who are rather monochrome whom it is tempting to take for granted, whom we actually find it very difficult to get interested in? People who maybe are desperate for us to take an interest in them, but who are afraid of closeness?

Sometimes dullness might be an unconscious defence, masking fantasies, although not necessarily as lurid as Quick's. They are only fantasies, but if only they could be talked about in therapy, they could perhaps provide pointers to how much the client wishes to be able to lead a more socially and personally fulfilling life; and pointing to directions the therapy might move.

Yet I also think about Quick's therapist, and those detectives, so eager to be involved with a headline case. And that they were so quick to judge, without really evaluating the evidence. What do I want to hear from my client? And do I seize upon it as soon as there is the slightest hint that it's what I want to hear?

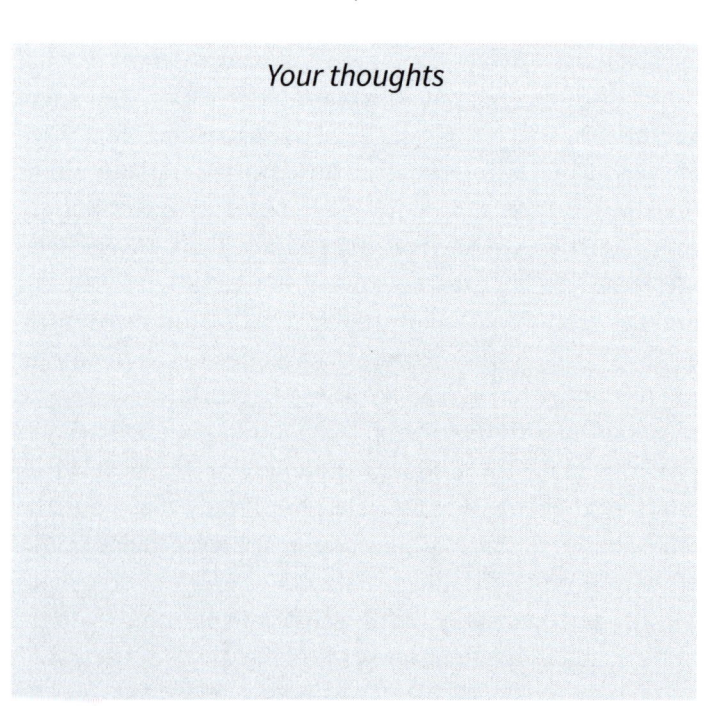

Your thoughts

12

A flexible core

Just as our bodies have a spine which in one sense holds us all together, so therapists need a spine, or perhaps (an image I prefer for reasons which will become clearer) a magnetic pole.

I use the image, not because I understand what a magnetic pole does, but because when we decide to train as a therapist, we are normally drawn, as if by a magnet, to a particular type of therapy, and that attraction normally stays with us in whatever direction we develop. This may be because it is the only training course available where we live; it may be because our own therapist, who has helped us so much, comes from that school of thought and practice; it may be because our impressions of the therapy are moulded by our admiration for one of its founders; or because it seems philosophically to suit us.

Whatever it is, I believe it is important to have that solid core, that pole that runs from north to south through our practice and our thinking, to which we return, especially when we are confused or needing to check out our understanding. It has the ability to support us and help us locate where we stand.

However, in most therapeutic approaches there are variations of thinking and practice, which are a sign of each one's richness as an approach. Here the image of the magnetic pole is again useful, because the pole shifts year by year—still performing the same function, but moving its location. So too we find that we may be drawn initially to Jung, but then find ourselves pulled slightly more towards one of the different branches of Jungian thought in preference to the others. Or to Freud, or Klein or to the Independent Group—or to attachment theory, self-psychology, intersubjective, modern relational theory, etc. We find ourselves adapting, partly because new situations suggest helpful and interesting alternative explanations or adaptations of practice, which used once in a particular context can then be applied in some others as well.

We even begin to cross over and check out systems which at one point, in our tribalism, we dismissed as not worth considering. Sometimes we find that similar concepts appear under different guises,[5] sometimes we find that it was not such a bad approach after all, only it missed

---

[5] See the *Core Concepts in Therapy* series I edited some years ago, published by the Open University Press.

something which we value; or that our own approach has missed something which we now come to value. Nevertheless, we remain held by the magnetism of our initial training and the ramifications of that approach as we deepen experience and knowledge. We begin to become our own person as a therapist; not eclectic, but integrating theory, practice, and what appeals to us as a person.

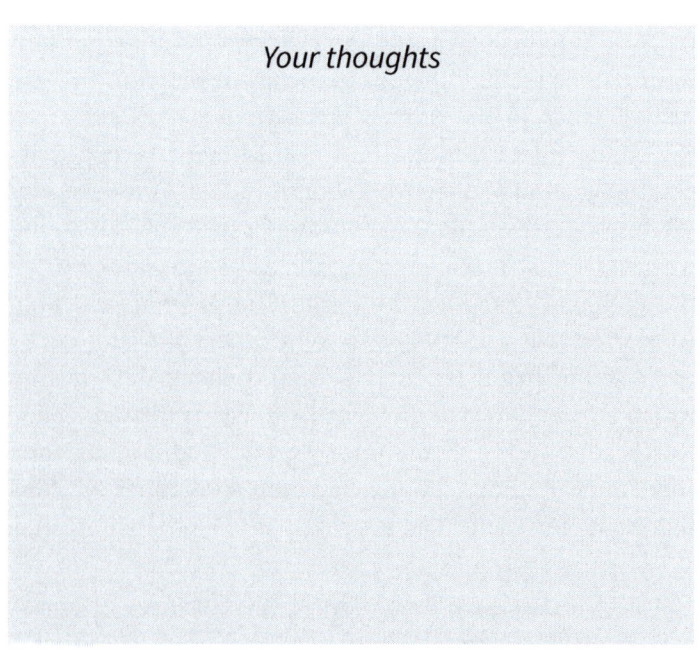

Your thoughts

13

My friend failure

It was odd. But misreadings often are odd. And what is odd is often informative. 'Therapeutic Failure', I read, as the title of a forthcoming conference. Oh no! It should have been 'Therapeutic Future'. Yet it seemed to me that a conference on therapeutic failure might be more interesting and certainly more relevant to my practice than one on the future of therapy.

'Failure has no friends', writes Arnold Goldberg.[6] That's because most of us find it very difficult to accept failure. Instead we tend to put the blame elsewhere: 'the client was not really motivated'; 'the client found it difficult to relate to me'; 'it was very difficult to be empathic towards him'—any reference to 'I' is banished from such excuses. Yet, as Goldberg continues, failure acts as an incentive to improvement; and if we are not prepared either to acknowledge our

---

[6] Goldberg, A. (2012). *The Analysis of Failure*. Hove: Routledge, p. 30.

failures or to find ways of addressing failure, we in fact fail ourselves.

Or as one of my own supervisors said, right at the start of my practice, 'We tend to teach from our successes, but we learn from our mistakes'. So I was pleased when asked at a question-and-answer session with students if I had ever made mistakes. 'Of course I have,' and I related a number of them, glaring errors, some of which seemed disastrous at the time, although most appeared to have been resolved in the sessions that followed. Or had they? Was that another way of dismissing my failure, to recall that the outcome was not in the end disastrous, even if it had set back the course of therapy for a while. Had I banished the failure by showing how in the end it was all to the good? It can be therapeutic, to fail; to acknowledge failure; and to work through it and to work it through. We show clients and ourselves that therapists are fallible; and that failures, disastrous though they seem, do not lead to disaster.

All of this is true, but it is only half the picture. What I realised as I looked back on my answer was that instead of fully embracing failure, I had to some extent sidelined it. Why didn't I realise, and why didn't I say that of course I had inevitably failed in many ways that I never knew about? That there must have been times when my clients never reacted visibly or verbally to my mistake; that I did not always reflect at the end of a session to see whether I might have made a mistake and therefore failed my client, because I was afraid to face failure, seeing it more as an enemy to my self-esteem than as a friend to my learning.

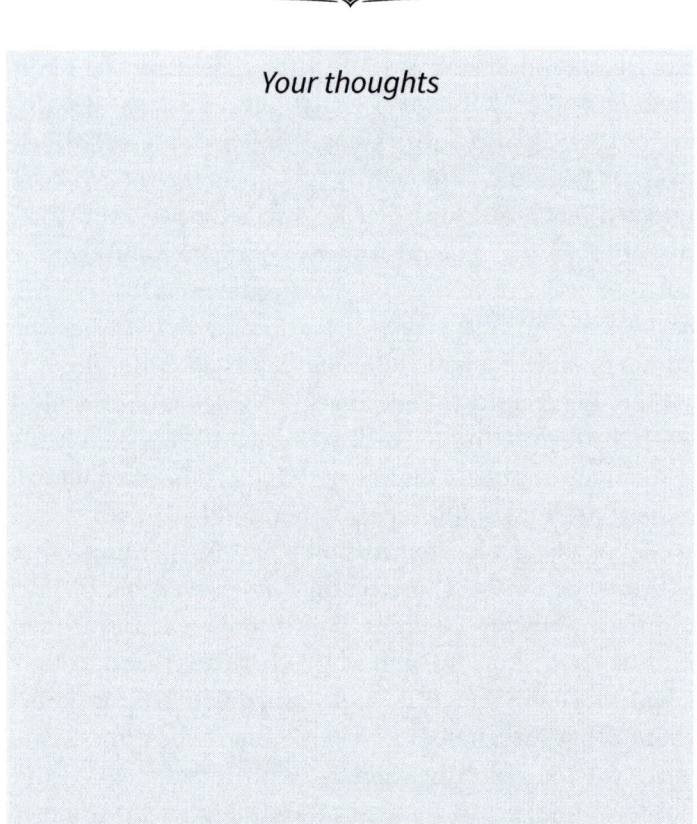

Your thoughts

14

Outbursts and inbursts

In *The Art of Unknowing* Stephen Kurtz suggests that therapists who are not constricted by a particular type of training will not be predictable in what they say. They will not know whether what they say is true or false, but they will exclaim OUTBURSTS (yes, the capitals are in the original).[7]

There is more to his argument than that, of course, but there is something in the word OUTBURSTS that is far from everything therapists are trained to be. And I contrast the suggestion with something the psychotherapist Peter Lomas[8] once said to me in conversation. Peter was describing how he had said something about himself to a patient

---

[7] Kurtz, S. (1989). *The Art of Unknowing: Dimensions of Openness in Analytic Therapy.* New York: Jason Aronson.

[8] Lomas, P. (2005). *Cultivating Intuition: A Personal Introduction to Psychotherapy.* London: Whurr.

which many therapists would have not revealed. 'But,' he said, 'I did not just blurt it out. I have a red light and a green light in my head, and there was no red light so I said it.'

There was no red light, but it seemed there was no green light either, yet he said what he had thought of saying, and he said that it did no harm. It seemed actually to help.

You can see the point. All the training and all the advice as to how to intervene as a therapist would appear to urge caution, especially in a situation where we do not know what to say. The safety of the client, or perhaps it is really the safety of the therapist, urges caution, something nondescript, an 'Um' or an 'Ah' perhaps, or repeating the last few of the client's words, essentially putting any more definite response on hold.

An OUTBURST suggests speaking without thinking, and not knowing what the effect on the client will be. I find it difficult to advocate that. But I do like the idea of what I would have to call an 'INBURST'—in other words, allowing myself to react spontaneously, inside my head, in my thoughts, not betraying by word or by facial or physical reaction, what my actual reaction or immediate thought or feeling is. That seems to me to be responding to a client as they are (which is what Kurtz also says); which is much more real than drawing up one of a number of standard, learned responses.

To be able to do that requires therapists to be themselves, and not putting on an act of being a therapist.

It's being genuine. But that does not mean being genuine behind a sort of therapeutic mask, because if we as therapists have honestly allowed ourselves to get in touch with every aspect of the way ordinary human beings can respond, that will mean that we are not shocked or even surprised by the INBURST: rather, aware that this particular reaction could be helpful once we have had the chance to process how to use it safely—waiting until the red light turns amber or, for the more cautious of us, turns green.

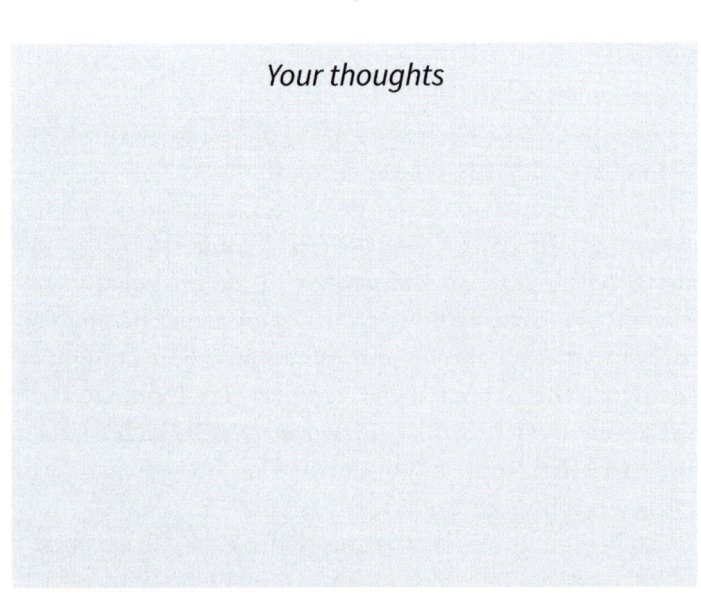

Your thoughts

15

Did you see… ?

It's not uncommon for any of us, talking with someone, to ask whether or not they saw such-and-such on the TV; or 'have you seen…?' a particular film; or 'have you read…?' And clients can ask such questions of their therapist; alternatively they may talk about a TV programme, a film, or a book.

I suggest it is probably wise not to answer the question 'Did you see?' positively. It is easier, of course, if we have to say 'No'; then it is natural to add, 'Tell me about it.' For the same reason, even if we have seen the film or know the book, we can say 'Yes, I saw that'; or 'Yes, I've read that too'; but it is probably better to deflect our response, which may inhibit the client's views: they may feel they don't need to say anything more.

We each react slightly differently to what we see or what we read. It is this that lies behind projection tests. We are all familiar with the inkblot cards—the Rorschach

Test—and some therapists may also have heard of the Thematic Apperception Test or the Object Relations Test, the latter consisting of twelve vague pictures, about which the respondent is asked to tell a story.

There are so-called standard ways of interpreting what the person responding to these tests sees. Where someone's interpretation differs from the most common results, that is often a significant pointer to an area which the psychologist might explore. But no such standard interpretations can exist for books, programmes, films, etc. (I'm not counting academic criticism here, although there too there can be wildly differing responses.) When we talk about what we have seen or what we have read, there is always an element of projecting our own meaning on to it. So, just as it is restrictive to try and interpret dreams by a set of standard meanings for the various symbols that feature in the dream story, what interests the therapist most is what *the client* makes of the programme, the book, the film they have referred to, of a piece of music they mention, or of a place they have visited.

Our response is better if it helps lead to an exploration: 'It sounds as if you saw it' or 'Have you just read it?' followed by 'What did you make of it?' That we too have read or seen it might lead to a conversation, but it risks influencing the client's voiced opinions. To respond without our own 'Yes' or 'No' is not to ignore the client's question. Instead we are giving clients the opportunity to say what they felt or what they thought. It does not preclude answering the original question later, after the client has had a full opportunity to talk.

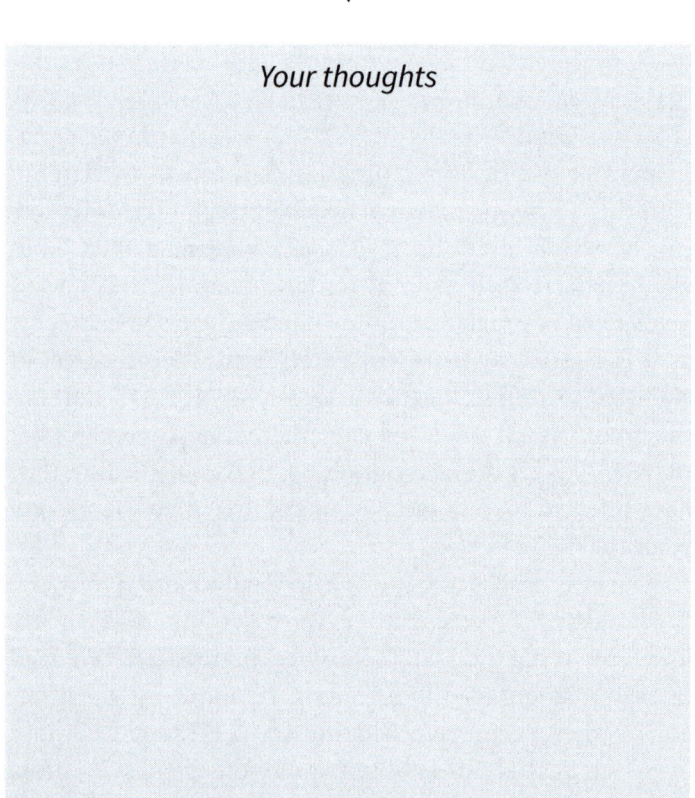

Your thoughts

16

As if …

Confucius was instructing his followers in offering gifts to the spirits and ghosts of their ancestors. The disciples asked him: 'But, Master, suppose there are no ghosts or spirits of the ancestors?' Confucius replied: 'Still act as if there are.'

'As if' is a fascinating little phrase. It can be used with scorn or mockery: 'As if!'—a pretty clear indication that you don't believe what you have been told. But it can be used more subtly, as Confucius does. Whether or not something is true, it is possible to act *as if* it is true, because that action is helpful whether or not the basis for it is true. In his case, it was good to remember your ancestors, whether or not there are any spirits.

Acting 'as if' something were true, when clearly it is not, is not always a sign of good thinking, and the results can be disastrous. Nevertheless, in the context of therapy those two little words are incredibly useful. Think of what we might say to clients: 'You are reacting to what I said *as if* I am your mother, who you tell me was constantly disapproving of all your efforts at school'; or 'You are concerned, it seems, that I might let you down, *as if* I was another of those so-called friends of yours who have turned their back on you.' We can react to others 'as if' they will respond a certain way. Clients can imagine what their therapist thinks about them, 'as if' they represent authoritarian figures in the client's past. These are instances where it can be very helpful for therapists to use the phrase, as a way of illustrating to clients how they are responding to situations, or choosing to act: 'as if' something is true, which, examined objectively, is not necessarily so.

There is a further way in which we might think about this little phrase. We probably do not need to refer to it in this sense in therapy, because it is something that applies all the time: that therapy itself is an 'as if' space, and the therapeutic hour is an 'as if' time. It is what the anthropologist might call a liminal, a sacred space. It is a place where fantasies can be spoken about, and possibilities voiced *as if* they happened or could happen. It is a place where the client can relate with the therapist *as if* the therapist were anyone the client wanted the therapist to be. It is *as if* the therapist and the therapy is a place where anything can happen, as if the normal conventions do not matter. In terms of actions, they do, but in terms of thought and speech they don't. The 'as if' can be a fiction, but it points to something real.

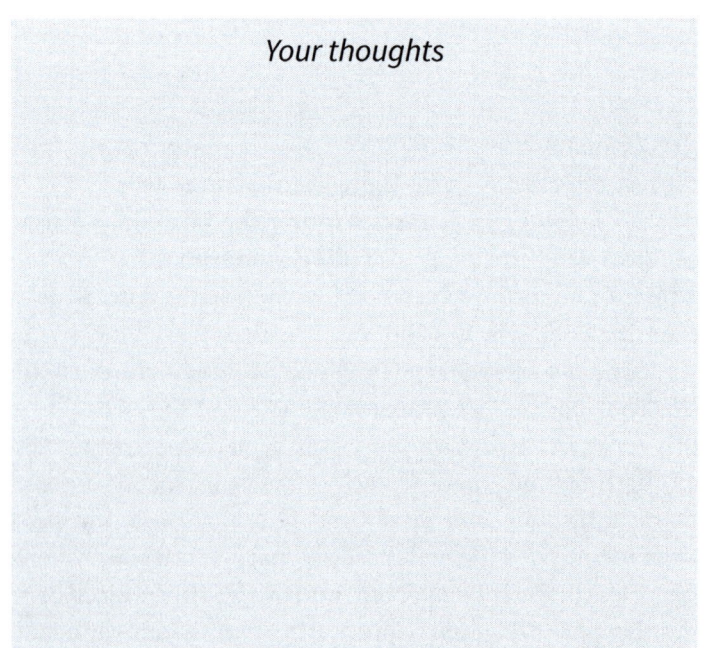

Your thoughts

17

Taking the flak

When a client is angry, either with you, for something you have either done or not done, whether or not you think it is deserved, or angry with someone else, but finding it difficult to hold back their anger, fearing they will explode and damage themselves and the other, then I sometimes am reminded of a scene in the 1950's film *The Dambusters.*[9]

Forgive me, because it's probably not your thing, but the image is for me a powerful one. In that film, the squadron leader, having already dropped his bouncing bomb, and not having yet breached the dam wall, is encouraging one of his other pilots as another plane makes its approach to the target. Knowing the amount of flak that was aimed at his own aircraft when he flew in to drop his bomb, the

---

[9] *The Dambusters* (1955), directed by Michael Anderson, music by Eric Coates.

squadron leader flies his plane across the top of the dam, to draw fire on himself, making it slightly safer for the next pilot to approach the bombing zone.

It's what therapists should be able to do: to take on themselves, for as long as necessary, the angry feelings that the client is expressing or wanting to express. We do this whether the anger is aimed at ourselves or not, trying to make it safer for the client. We may ask whether the client is feeling angry 'here' and 'with me'. Or rather more confidently, we may actually suggest to the client that 'I think you may well be feeling angry with me too'. Indeed that may well be so, that we have actually said or done the wrong thing, or not said or done the right thing, and perhaps not realised it. It may help clients to address the mistakes we have made, our lack of understanding, or a response that we got wrong. Acknowledging our fallibility is another of those personal qualities we need to have, on a par with being empathic and genuine.

A client's response may well be that 'of course' they are not angry with us. And that's OK. There's no need then to go on pushing that line: either it doesn't strike the client that way, or the client is afraid to admit that that is what they feel. But we have sown the idea, that it's OK to talk about being angry with us, that we are able to take it, that it will not kill us: that being able to express angry feelings is just as much part of the therapeutic process as anything else. In fact, it's a darn sight less risky for us to take the flak than it was for that squadron leader when he sought to protect his fellow pilot. And he survived.

Your thoughts

18

A sprinkling of CPD

A therapist was reflecting upon her life's work, comparing how it had been in the service she had been working in all her life in earlier years and how it was at her point of leaving it.[10] It was a passing remark, but one that stuck out as being illustrative of the difference between the earlier and the later time. She explained that over the years she had learned so much from working with her clients ('wisdom gleaned from those who went before'), and that it was this which really made the difference in her work; together with (and this was the phrase that struck me) 'a sprinkling of what I have learned from theory and research'.

There really is no substitute for it: that is, for the work itself, for each of the five hours she used to spend each day,

---

[10] Dr Tara Porter, *The Guardian*, Wednesday 7 December 2022.

five days a week, working with her clients. It was where many of us in the early days also learned our craft. There was no 'CPD' in those days: or rather there was nothing but CPD, because the way we developed professionally was continuously learning from our clients, as well as from the conversations we had in supervision. And when we came to supervise others ourselves, there were not even courses to learn how to do it. Again, we learned by doing it.

Of course, it would be antediluvian to deny the value of what is on offer these days, the shelves of books, the plethora of courses, the research that can inform practice. But how much time should it take up, compared to the amount of practice, which is the best training ground of them all? What a great word it is—'practice': because that is what we do, although as a verb we spell that with an 's': 'I practise as a therapist'. Yet 'practice' in the sense of working away at learning, at improving, at gaining confidence in what we have learned for ourselves—that is also what we do. We don't 'practice' on clients, but we practise with them, and in doing so we 'practice' our skills, always learning, often refining, sometimes finding for ourselves what works best with this or that person.

And if we have to show evidence of CPD as a paper exercise, and attend for so many hours to learn new tricks, can we regard those hours as 'sprinklings' of theory, research, and practical methods? And the core of what we are doing day by day as the real continuing professional development?

Your thoughts

19

The way

It is perhaps the central image that we associate with Buddhism, Taoism, and no doubt in other religions: the Way. And it is central to the idea of the Way that each person must find it for themselves. There is no easy way to find the Way, let alone travel along it.

Let me bring the image a little nearer to being a therapist. We of course do not, or try not to, give directions for the individual client's way forward, or even backward. We can understand the words of a Tibetan master who says: 'Showing others the path / When you don't know the way / Harms yourself and others'.[11]

Our intention, no doubt, is to accompany, or attempt to accompany the client along their way, and to do that involves the capacity to empathise with what the client may

---

[11] Heruka, T. (2010). *The Life of Milarepa*, A. Quintman (Trans.). London: Penguin Books.

be going through. It is less difficult to do this when what the client is feeling overlaps with our own experiences, or with what we have learned from closely following the experiences of others with whom we have previously trodden the way. But can we really be empathic if what we are hearing or witnessing is far removed from our own experience? How can we be sure that even if there is some overlap between the client's experience and our own, there are not circumstances which make our empathic responses feel OK to us, but only marginally touch the client's?

Empathy is central to counselling practice; perhaps for some therapists the only way to be alongside a client. But empathy comes from knowing the client, and if we do not know enough about the client and the client's way, then we risk harming ourselves and them: ourselves because we believe ourselves to be more empathic than we actually are; and clients because we are falling short in supporting them as they find their way.

The lesson from this is that before being empathic, we need to learn from the client, and need to learn to distinguish our clients from ourselves. We really need to be saying more often than we do: 'Can you help me understand what you are going through (or, what you have been through)?' Perhaps we might also be saying, in intention if not in actual words: 'Can you take me into that dark, that lonely place, so I may be able to feel it with you?' We need to travel that way with them, re-treading with them the path that has brought them to our door. We speak, then, closer to their experience rather than simply our own.

Your thoughts

20

A cigar is a cigar is a cigar

There is a tendency—a strong tendency we might even say—for those therapists who espouse a psychoanalytic or psychodynamic tradition to want to analyse everything. And there is nothing wrong with that, as long as it is not pressed too hard, especially upon the client. And as long as we can just once in a while accept that a spade is a spade, and is what the client has called it.

It was something that Freud encountered. He was someone who was always looking behind things to find what they stood for, notably in connection with dreams, symptoms, and everyday mistakes. Having dismissed the old-fashioned but popular dream books of his day, which listed what images in dreams stood for, Freud (or perhaps it was those who followed him) seems to have set up his own dream interpretations. But when he was asked on his visit to America (although it is probably an apocryphal story) what it meant that he loved cigars so much, he replied, 'A cigar is a cigar is a cigar.'

It's a good joke. It may also be a valid point to make for those who want to criticise Freud for seemingly analysing everything. Such a response, were it ever made, would not have satisfied some of his early followers. One, for example, writes that 'the cigar reminds us of the male organ burning with desire';[12] while another writes that smoking a cigar is a return to the mother's breast.[13]

Yet, if we pursue the story a little further, of course it meant something, which Freud would eventually have to have admitted. For one thing, it meant a good smoke; for another, it seems as if it might have helped him to cope with a heavy workload, and calmed him. And that would have been worth talking about. It's not necessarily the deeper meanings that are the most significant.

Symbols are of course important. They do carry meaning, although it is necessary to remember that they carry different meanings for different people. Everyday objects as much as pictures, dreams, stories, all carry meaning. A cigar (or an e-cigarette) is not just a cigar, but it does not

---

[12] Ferenczi, S. (1922). The symbolism of the bridge. *International Journal of Psychoanalysis*, 3: 163–168, p. 167.
[13] Boehm, F. (1930). The feminity-complex in men. *International Journal of Psychoanalysis*, 11: 444–469, p. 452.

have to become something as simple (for the analyst) as a penis or a breast. Anything we or the client bring to the session has a potential story to tell. But it is not always the one we imagine.

Your thoughts

21

Great expectations

There's quite a difference between objectives and expectations. Objectives—which a therapist may want to discuss or even plan with a client—aim to be realistic goals for their work together: what the client would like to achieve and what the therapist believes might be practical and possible. Expectations depend much more upon wishes and fears—conscious and unconscious—and are very often not realistic. Think, for example, of situations where you have had high hopes, but the reality has led to disappointment. Or the more pleasant opposite, where your expectations are very low, and you have been more than relieved when they turned out better than you thought possible. High expectations of therapy, of a therapist, or even of a client can often lead to disappointment and disillusion; low expectations may sometimes result in pleasant surprises.

It's worth thinking about our own expectations of ourselves as therapists, and what we imagine at times we can or cannot achieve; and challenging our assumptions about our skills. Equally, we always need to think, especially in the opening sessions with a new client, of what that person's expectations are of us and of what they hope therapy can achieve. Some of their expectations are that as therapists we know all the answers, or that a session or two will set things back on course; or indeed that therapy is probably worth trying, but there isn't much hope that it will do any good. Sometimes these expectations are expressed openly, but more often that not there are assumptions which a client can have: wishes or fears, that are not spoken and may even not be clear to the client.

These expectations are in a sense illusory, at least in that they remain to be tested; and that is not necessarily easily done. They cannot be altered simply by rational discussion. The negative expectation that the therapist is going to judge me, even if it's not obvious, doesn't evaporate just like that; indeed, the assumption may need to be tested time and again, and only change through experience not reassurance. Even then, it will lurk ready to appear again at any moment. The positive expectation that if we go on long enough we will change may also have to be challenged, not through argument, but through gradual disillusion.

Then, of course, we need to be alert to what disillusion means: having to relinquish high expectations is like having to let go of something precious; indeed, high expectations may have come about as compensation for earlier disappointments. It is different, of course, when low expectations are proved wrong, where it is good to share in the discovery that therapy is more helpful than was thought. However, ultimately, expectations, as distinct from objectives, don't get us very far, and may be more of an impediment than an incentive.

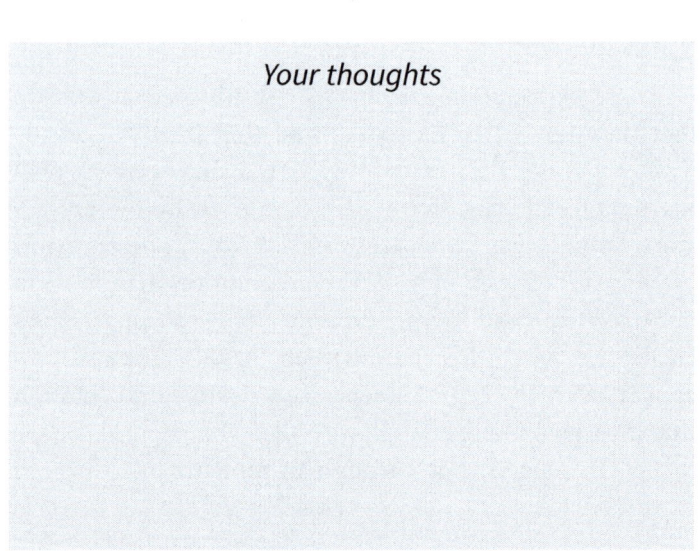

Your thoughts

22

What do you do?

That seems like an easy question to answer, when someone you meet asks 'What do you do?' 'Oh, I'm a psychotherapist' or 'I'm a counsellor'. But our enquirer pushes us further: 'Yes, but what do you *do*?'

Well, what *do* you do? How would you explain?

Are you an expert on psychological disorders? Is that it? Or is it simpler than that? 'I encourage people to talk with me … to unload their worries … to look into their upbringing and see how it relates to their present situations … etc.' You know the sort of thing, since you've probably had to answer the question of what you do several times. You may even have felt the question to be rather threatening, as if what you actually do is really not easy to describe. You come away feeling you have not done justice to your profession. It's all rather airy-fairy, and you may be tempted to fall back on research, or on technical explanations that show you can't do this sort of thing without a thorough training in psychotherapeutic techniques. 'I investigate the unconscious' might shut your enquirer up! Actually, sometimes just saying what you do does shut them up!

Suppose you were an artist, or a writer. 'What do you do?' 'Oh … I paint'; or 'Well … I write'. That's clear enough, and if your enquirer asks what you paint or what you write, then you may describe generally what you have done, or what you are doing. Your enquirer will have understood what you do perfectly and be more interested, not in how you do it, but in the subjects that interest you. The enquirer is less likely to ask what techniques you use in painting, or how you go about writing a book. And surely therapy is rather like being an artist or a writer. You really don't know what your client is going to bring to the session, and you have to work with raw material—raw in more than one sense—each new session. You draw upon your experience, your creativity, your humanity, and of course from time to time upon your knowledge, though your knowledge (that is what was taught in your training) is probably a small part of the mix.

'What I *actually* do?' may be inappropriate to describe to the enquirer in the context of a casual conversation; but is a rather good question to ask ourselves, in the quiet of the consulting room. If I can identify what I actually do, then I may be able to pinpoint what I do well, and where I need to develop as a therapist.

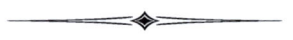

Your thoughts

23

Fears and wishes

I am always pleased to find examples of where dynamic therapy and behaviour therapy speak with a similar voice. I came across such an example when I was checking what Freud suggested about phobias. He explained them as projections of wishes that were repressed, together with fears of punishment for those unconscious wishes. It is as if unconscious anxieties are attached to a particular object, which itself represents a threat to be avoided; so that allows the person to 'get on' with living, as long as they can avoid that specific danger.

Dynamic therapy has generally found phobias very difficult to work with, and non-analytic treatments, such as behavioural therapy, are often recommended.

I then found a different explanation of phobias, also from a psychoanalytic perspective.[14] The writer believes

---

[14] Moraitis, G. (1991). Phobias and the pursuit of novelty. *Psychoanalytic Inquiry*, *11*: 296–315.

that phobias arise from fear of the unknown. This makes a lot of sense. Most young children seem to have little fear, and are ready to explore anything new that attracts their attention and interest. It is the calm presence of their carers and awareness of their capacity to contain fear that helps the child build up a confidence in themselves as well. An illustration from Winnicott: 'A child is playing in the garden. An aeroplane flies low overhead—you hold the child close to yourself, and the child uses the fact that you are not scared beyond recovery'.[15] Phobias are therefore not about a specific unconscious wish that has to be avoided at all cost; but more about a less-than-confident self, perhaps not having had carers who were able to contain early anxieties about the unknown.

This is not a comprehensive explanation, but it suggests the therapist is not so interested in the object of the phobia and what it stands for, as in the value of talking about the unknown fear or fears. The author's recommendation (and here is the parallel with the behaviour therapist) is that where there is a phobia, the therapist's approach is to gradually encourage it to be talked about, time and time again, until it begins to subside, although it is unlikely it will disappear altogether. The unknown gradually becomes more familiar and less threatening, since it is held within the

---

[15] Davis, M., & Wallbridge, D. (1981). *Boundary and Space*. London: Karnac, p. 99.

safety of the therapeutic process. It is the calm presence of the therapist, who in a metaphorical sense holds the client close to themselves and contains their own fears when dangerous thoughts and feelings 'fly low overhead', which gradually loosens some of the most crippling fears of the unknown.

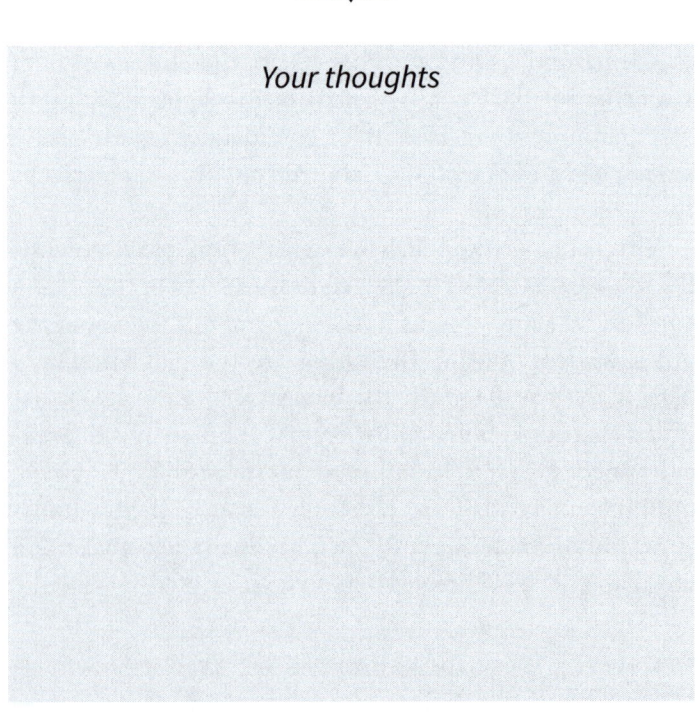

Your thoughts

24

Apologies

It's amazing how many therapists, who have been hauled before a disciplinary panel having had a complaint made against them, did not know how to say 'Sorry' to their client when they made some sort of mistake. It is as if the therapist is caught by a retaliatory mechanism, which means that if the client criticises a therapist, the therapist becomes defensive, rather than discussing what they have apparently done wrong and how it might be worked through.

Of course we make mistakes as therapists; and if that mistake upsets the client, it seems rather encouraging that they protest. There is no need to have to defend yourself when someone takes offence, even if their offence is triggered by taking things the wrong way. If the client takes something I have said or done, or not said or not done, as in some way a personal insult, or as a damaging wound, surely my first response is to help them express what they feel; and then to look at what they think about it. I stress what they *think*, as well as what they feel, because sometimes once the feeling has been expressed, thinking about it can show that it was all a bit of a storm in a teacup, nevertheless showing up a sensitive spot.

Should we apologise in the first instance, even if we think we did nothing wrong? It might be a way of creating a space in which feelings and reactions can be examined, on both sides. We can certainly say that we are sorry that the client feels aggrieved. There is always the possibility that the client has got it wrong: that we did not say what the client thought we said. Or that the client is particularly delicate in some areas—often to implied criticism. It's easy enough for any of us to get angry when we are anxious, and no one seems to be able to help. If a client complains, the right response is not to get defensive, but to explore what we have done, or not done, what we have said or not said; what that feels like to the client; and what it means for the client. It doesn't matter if the client has got it wrong: we don't have to justify ourselves. 'The customer is always right', they say, and for the time being we can respond as if the client is right, and as if we are in the wrong. Later there may be an opportunity, when both sides have calmed down, to look at it from a different angle.

The point is that we may have got it wrong without realising it—and even without the client realising it. We do what we can, and we draw upon our experience as fully as we can, but we are not omniscient. We can and do make mistakes.

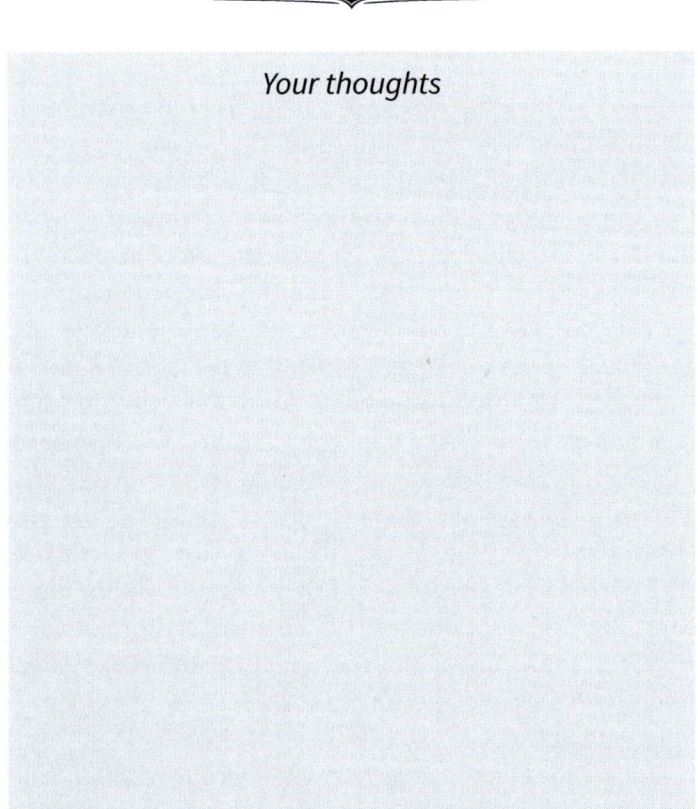

Your thoughts

25

The ambivalence of the therapist

Do you enjoy being a therapist? Or is 'enjoy' the wrong word? Perhaps not, because there are clients with whom it is a joy to work, and there are clients whom a therapist really does not look forward to seeing. But is that solely to do with different types of client? At first that may seem to be the case, but it is worth looking a little deeper.

I suspect that the people we enjoy working with most are those who are open to the approach we value ourselves, the one that suits our own personality. It is interesting to think about something Winnicott said to the psychotherapist and author Harry Guntrip. It was towards the end of Guntrip's analysis with Winnicott: 'I'm good for you but you're good for me. Doing your analysis is almost the most reassuring thing that happens to me. The chap before you makes me think I'm no good at all'.[16] We might suspect that one of the reasons that Winnicott felt good about working with him was because he was a good talker (rather too much, according to Winnicott) and that he worked hard on trying to delve deeper into himself. We don't know what it was about 'the chap before you' that made Winnicott feel no good at all. But we will probably understand the sentiment.

So, at first glance, the people we enjoy working with are those who make us feel good as therapists, and perhaps even more make us feel good about ourselves.

They are 'suitable clients' who tick all the boxes, those who fit the descriptions of the clients we should be taking on. And those we don't look forward to seeing, they are the clients who don't fit the criteria, although these will to some extent be different clients for different therapists.

Yet it is not as simple an equation as that: the danger is that with those whom we enjoy working with we slip into a rather collusive relationship. For instance, we know that Guntrip talked a huge amount in his sessions, and it is possible that he did so because he dreaded feeling abandoned

---

[16] Guntrip, H. (1996). My experience of analysis with Fairbairn and Winnicott: How complete a result does psychoanalytic therapy achieve? *International Journal of Psychoanalysis*, *77*: 739–754, p. 750.

in the silence. We know that Winnicott said to Guntrip that he (Guntrip) had 'always been able to give more than to take'. The 'good client' can lull us into a false sense of how well we are working.

And one of the dangers in working with those we enjoy seeing is that we fail to see those aspects that might make us feel 'no good at all'.

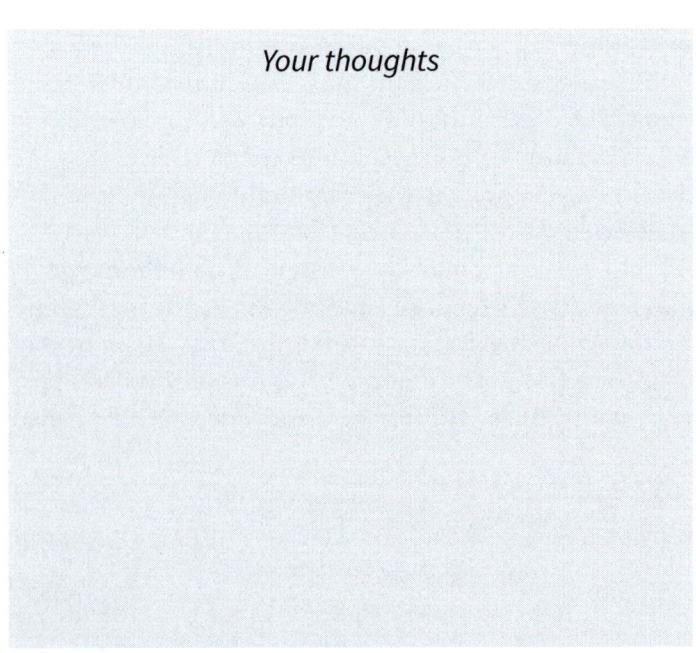

Your thoughts

26

The ambivalence of the therapist—further thoughts

'The chap before you makes me think I'm no good at all'.[17] What might Winnicott's patient have been like to make him feel he was no good at all? It is difficult to imagine the man Winnicott wrote about, the one who repelled him initially, but whom he was eventually able to tell that he had become lovable.[18] Difficult because the thing about that patient was that he seems to have aroused massive negative feelings in others, and that fact at the very least must have made him interesting to work with. A challenge, if nothing else.

---

[17] Guntrip, H. (1996). My experience of analysis with Fairbairn and Winnicott: How complete a result does psychoanalytic therapy achieve? *International Journal of Psychoanalysis*, *77*: 739–754, p. 750.
[18] Winnicott, D. W. (1975). *Through Paediatrics to Psycho-Analysis*. London: Hogarth, p. 196.

It may be the challenging client with whom it is difficult to say we enjoy being a therapist. Then there are the clients who are 'sent' and who lack motivation to use therapy for themselves. Some of those keep on attending, perhaps because they feel forced to, perhaps because there is something about us which just about keeps them in contact, hanging on by a thread. And there are those who (sadly) are rather boring, at least in their presentation, where we may wonder what it is that stirs in their depths.

It is inevitable that our work as therapists has its ups and downs, that it involves a mixture of people, some of whom we look forward to seeing and some of whom we don't. The important thing with all of them is not to lose sight of the therapeutic task, which is to reflect on what we are seeing and feeling, and to reflect on what we are not seeing and feeling. That reflection includes our own experience with the client, whether that experience gives us a clue to how others perceive the client, and how the client perceives themselves.

Is it possible that when as a therapist we feel 'no good at all' that this is precisely what our client is sitting there feeling? If we are feeling repelled by the client, is the client keeping us at a distance because the client cannot allow us too close? If we have negative feelings about a client, may the client also have those negative feelings towards us? If we are feeling bored by a client, what seems to compel that person to keep anything interesting or exciting at bay?

These could be the situations where we have to develop and draw upon skills we did not know we had.

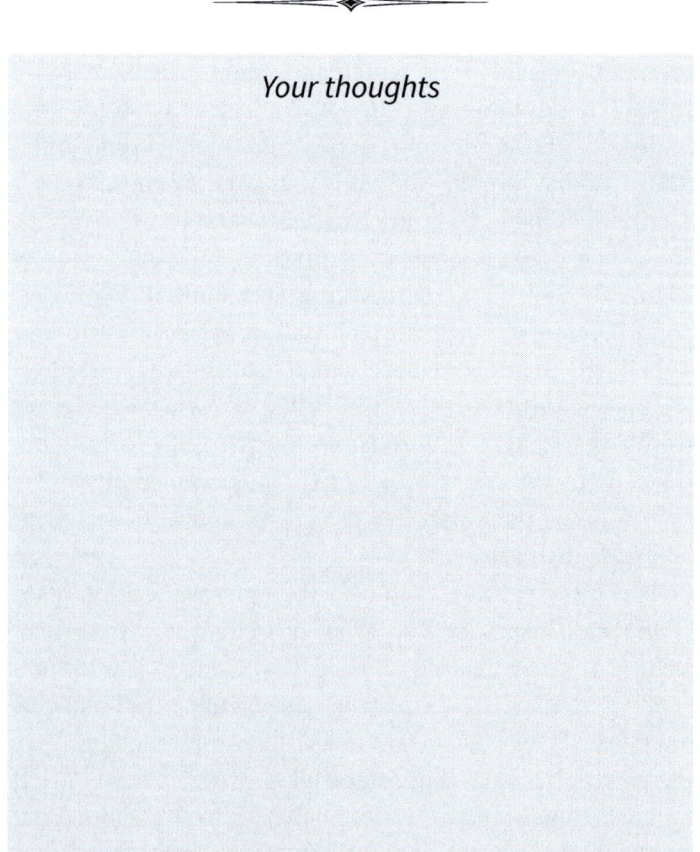

Your thoughts

27

Let be

It must be difficult filming wildlife; having to let nature takes its course, and not intervening when an animal or bird is in trouble. And there is a similar difficulty for therapists when a decision has to be made whether or not to intervene; or more accurately, how to intervene when the client is troubled.

There are many reasons people become therapists, but two of the reasons that are probably near the top of the list are firstly, because of a concern to help others; and secondly, because of an interest in what makes us tick, and how different experiences and their effects on us might be understood. Likewise, there are many reasons why people seek therapy, probably the top two being that they want to feel better; and that they want to understand why they feel the way they do.

In therapy there are times which are just like those agonising moments on wildlife documentaries, when we wish someone would step in and help. But they can't. And we can't. We have to let it be. Then there are times when the therapist has to decide whether to step in and rescue the client, and whether to stay with the client in their pain and suffering. The therapist might even wish someone could step in and help the therapist as well.

On the whole the therapist is a supporter, but not a rescuer. There are many situations where it would be very unwise to rescue the client, since it would ultimately resolve nothing: giving the client money (although Freud did that sometimes!); offering to write or in some other way intervene in a dispute outside therapy (although occasionally there is good reason to confirm someone is in therapy); or, depending on your orientation, offering physical comfort, which, even if appropriate, needs to be handled very carefully.

More often than not we have to let be. Not simply because it is important that people are allowed to express their feelings (particularly if they are upset, hurt, angry, etc.). We still need to gauge how helpful it is to stay with their pain and when it becomes counterproductive. Nevertheless, we cannot take away another's pain. If we have to intervene, we remember that the pain is still there, not yet plumbed to its depth.

It's easier to try and help than it is to let be. Yet letting be, standing by while allowing and even encouraging what hurts to be felt and voiced, can lead to a calm space where it becomes possible to talk more dispassionately again, and to address the causes, and possible resolutions, of the pain.

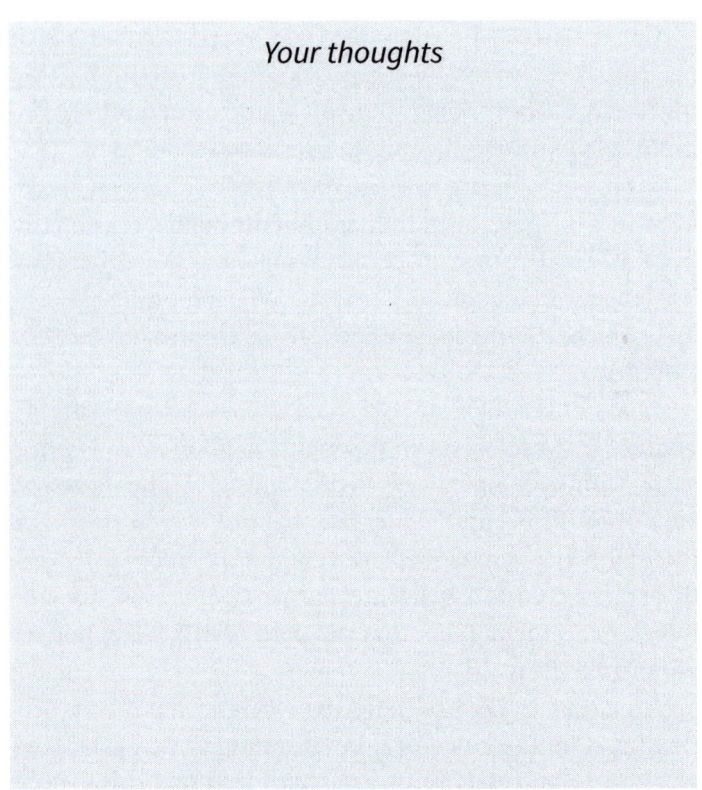

Your thoughts

28

Silence

Silence can be golden, but it can also feel very leaden. It has many different meanings in the therapeutic situation, and it can reflect many different moods. It has been described, in relation to long silences, as being defensive—perhaps it is difficult to speak because of shame, about what the client might be thinking of saying. Perhaps the silence is controlling, since refusing to speak is an attempt to make the therapist take the initiative. Or is the silence hostile or sulky, trying to make the therapist feel uncomfortable? It may be a passive–aggressive expression of anger towards the therapist or the process. It may even be revenge, countering the silence of the therapist.

On the other hand, silence is an opportunity, especially where none of the possibilities in the last paragraph apply. It gives time for both therapist and client to reflect upon what has passed between them in the preceding part of the session. Particularly poignant or distressing occasions in therapy need a period of calm to process what has happened, to ponder what has been said, and to process feelings that have been evoked. Both therapist and client need to learn when it is more helpful to keep quiet than to press a point too hard. It is especially helpful when therapists can allow themselves space, when the silence of the session allows them to monitor what they are themselves feeling, and whether what they are feeling mirrors what the client is experiencing.

There are many ways, if a silence is too long and becoming awkward and uncomfortable, for the therapist to intervene: we can ask how the client is feeling (if we cannot perceive it ourselves); or comment on the silence that has fallen and wonder what the client has been thinking. But a long and unproductive silence presents another opportunity, which is to move towards an exploration of what the client's experience of communication was like in their family of origin. Was silence a predominant feature? Did family members talk much to each other, especially when relationships became tense? Was it difficult to talk about problems or painful experiences with other family members? And what are the client's present relationships like: do they talk much to friends and current family? Some families are very quiet, or only skim the surface in their conversations, and some friendships only work because of a shared interest. Any of these pathways can lead back in turn to how it feels in the present therapeutic relationship. This provides something of a marker to know how to respond when long silences fall in later sessions, and whether these silences reflect any of the past or present situations the client has described.

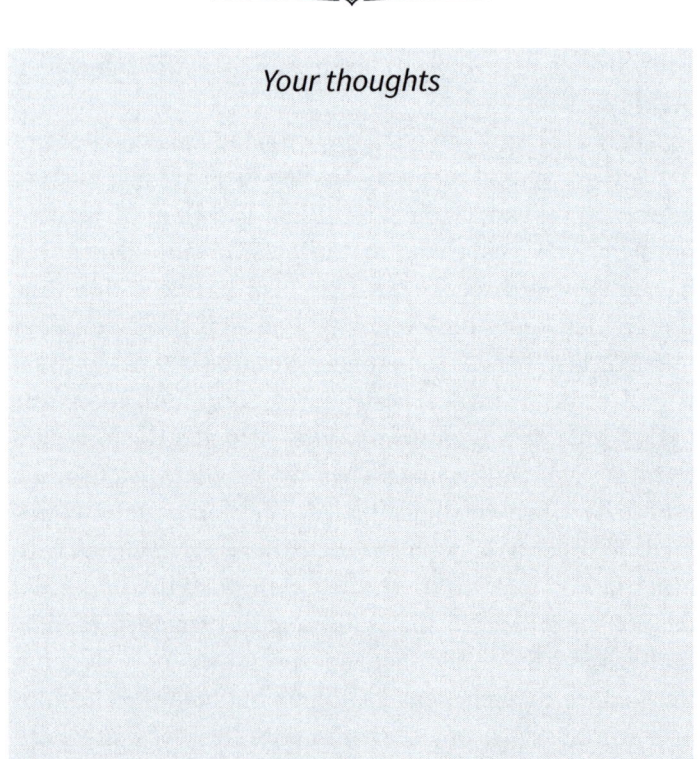

Your thoughts

29

Outcomes and goals

What do you hope to achieve for your clients as a therapist?

Freud had various goals for analysis at different times of his life: first, it was translating neurotic misery into common unhappiness. That is not bad as an outcome, suitably modest, and difficult enough to achieve even with such a low objective. No one can expect a smooth passage through life, and finding a way of approaching and accepting life's ups and downs helps. Freud later thought that it was about making the unconscious conscious. An analyst tells the story of a new patient who fiercely proclaimed that she was into consciousness-raising, and asked the therapist what he was into. Stumped for a while by the forcefulness of the question, he said '*Unconsciousness* raising'. Interesting, but surely not enough? Yet the patient's question was apt: 'What are you into?'

Freud's last definition of a goal was 'Where id was, there ego shall be': a plea for a thought out, realistic approach to meeting the many and varied situations in life. I suspect many would set their goals as being more multi-faceted than that. There is also the straightforward goal that the client should feel, when leaving therapy, that it has been of benefit to them: the value of this goal that it is not defined at the outset. Given that clients need to spend a lot to undergo this process, we hope that there is at least some benefit. But I don't think that is sufficient.

Others have come up with alternative outcomes. While it does not appeal to the radical, we could suggest that therapy is helping people towards normality, if we only knew what normality is. Many years ago, I remember a thread in an online discussion forum that discussed how psychological well-being might be described. As therapists, we more readily look at what is not working for a person rather than what would be the signs of a healthy balanced individual. The list of positive outcomes grew and grew, yet it seemed impossible to come up with a neat definition of normality.

Yet another suggestion is the opposite, that as therapists we are in the business of helping people accept their individuality or their uniqueness, which may mean that they may not precisely conform to what is thought to be the definition of a healthy individual. Such a definition of good outcome has some similarity to the view that it is the client who sets the agenda, although I believe therapists have theirs, and they are part of the mix. It is not just about self-acceptance, but enabling people to develop their own unique characteristics for their benefit, and perhaps (because your goal may include a societal dimension) for the benefit of others.

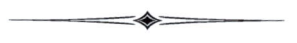

Your thoughts

30

The response

He arrived on time and sat down comfortably. He started to tell me about his week, and I looked for some connecting theme in what he was saying but could not yet see one. In any case it was too early for that. I wondered which aspect of his week I might take up, but could not make up my mind, and so kept quiet.

He talked on, an interesting story about an incident at work. I could make nothing of it, and I felt I was not functioning very well. Was this telling me something about his week too? I couldn't see any connection. I only responded with 'mms' and 'ahs', and could not get into anything he was saying.

I asked a question, for want of anything else to say. I still could make neither head nor tail of anything that might spark a helpful intervention from my side. This was one of those days, it seemed, when I couldn't grasp anything, although I sensed that the fault lay in me and not in him.

I told myself that this wasn't a fault, and that I should stop blaming myself; but I was still mulling over the difficulty I was having in saying anything helpful. While listening with one ear to him, I was more troubled listening to myself. What was I doing? Or rather, why was I not doing anything? Anything I did say seemed empty and rather useless, although he would start describing another situation, which he related in some detail. He reflected on what he had been saying, while I felt as if I ought to be giving more encouragement than I was able to. I tried hard to connect what he was saying with what I was feeling, but again it got me nowhere. I was feeling very stuck, more concerned by now about my own lack of response than thinking about what might be useful to say.

What might my client be telling me about himself and me? That took me nowhere. I wondered whether there was something defensive about him, but that didn't feel right. He was speaking very freely. By now I wanted the session to end because I was getting nowhere. I was twisted up in knots and failing to attend to him. The only positive thing about me that day was that I was able to sit more calmly than I felt inside and to maintain eye contact with him. At least I was outwardly relaxed.

We came to the end of the session. I said that time was up, that I looked forward to seeing him next week. It all felt rather empty as I said it.

His response: 'Oh, yes. I'll see you again next week. I look forward to it. A very helpful session. Thank you.'

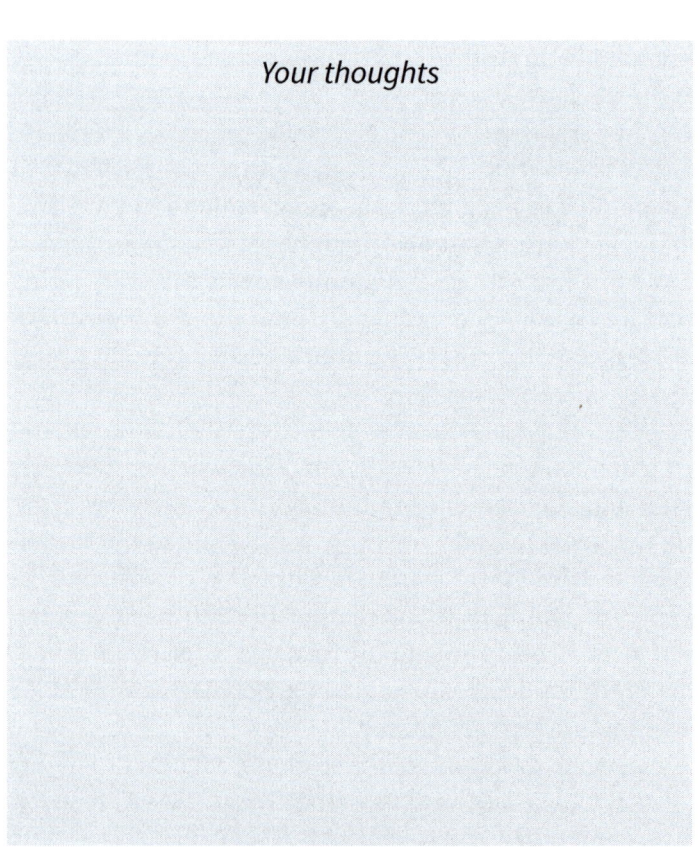

Your thoughts

31

Niggles

There's a word for that sensation when you cannot get a certain musical phrase out of your head: the one you keep humming, the one that silently buzzes around in your consciousness: the earworm. Rather similar is a niggle, although by this I don't mean something you feel sore about or want to complain about. I mean more a word or a phrase which strikes you, and which you can't quite get hold of. Now why did that word or phrase occur to you like that?

It's an irritant in one way, though not necessarily an unpleasant one. It's rather like that feature of crime stories where the detective says, having viewed the scene, that there was something they felt or saw which wasn't quite right, but they're not sure what it was; or that a certain object stuck in their memory; or that an object they would expect to be there wasn't. Much later, when everyone is stumped and you still do not know 'whodunit', the detective suddenly sees what it was, and what the significance is, and everything falls into place. Crime solved.

Freud used the image of the detective to illustrate how understanding a person's condition is not as straightforward as a detective coming on a crime scene and immediately seeing a photo of the criminal. No, there are all sorts of minor clues, which the detective has to look for and gradually piece together, trying to identify the offender.

Such niggles can be something a client said, or did not say, which you are left with after the session, although it's not always something that you registered at the time. Out of the blue there's this niggle, and you can't get it out of your mind. It's no good trying to think about it systematically, because it's not a straightforward problem that you can sit down and think about, or discuss in supervision. It's more like an irritant, an itch that doesn't go away however much you scratch it.

It's probably best not to give too much attention to what niggles. Your unconscious mind picks up things your conscious mind ignores. Your unconscious needs to work it out before you do. You won't get to understand your niggle by looking back at your notes or trying to work out your associations to it. Let it go on niggling. Be patient. Something has lodged in your mind, so just wait. You won't forget it if it's important. Sleep on it. At some point it will be there again, perhaps in a later session; and then you will see and understand why it niggled in the first place. Even if it does not unlock everything, it means something and eventually gives you something to work with.

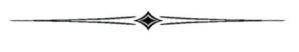

Your thoughts

32

There's always a flip side

'Ambivalent' is a curious word. It often means that someone is undecided, not sure which choice to make. But it has a more precise meaning in psycho-dynamic terminology. Ambivalence is the holding together of two contrary aspects, most often referred to as being able to hold together love and hate for the same object, or the same person. It is not (as in the common definition) 'I don't know whether or not I love him or hate him', but 'I love *and* hate him'. Not either/or, but both/and. Not necessarily in equal measure but always having the capacity to recognise love and hate towards the same object.

That makes me wonder whether ambivalence stretches far wider than love and hate, and whether there is often, if not always, a flip side to our feelings and perhaps to our views as well. It makes me wonder whether we ought as therapists to be more alert to the possibility of the contrary view or feeling which the client is expressing, and whether and how we might be able to introduce that into the mix. It often applies to the whole business of coming to therapy itself. Someone wants help, but at the same time does not want it, because of what it might involve. A client has positive feelings for you, but does not recognise their more negative feelings, when you are in fact just as withholding as you are giving of yourself.

Someone may be very excited about a forthcoming engagement, but are they also anxious. Excitement may be the opposite of fear, just as Freud suggested that fear masks a wish. There may be something in his idea—or there may not! Someone may be very anxious about facing a new situation, but at the same time may be looking forward to what benefit it might bring.

Jung is pretty good about all this, since he posits various opposites—anima and animus, introvert and extravert, thinking and feeling (alternatively, reason and emotion), sensing and intuition. Where there is only one side which is obvious, we might wonder what has happened to the other side. It may be split off, so that instead of two contrary views or feelings being attributed to the same object, they are split on to quite distinct objects.

Much is asked of the therapist. It is indeed easy to be drawn into one side of a client's views and feelings, particularly where they are strong views or intense feelings, without finding space to wonder what the flip side is. Perhaps one of the tasks of the therapist is to hold the other side in mind, perhaps even carry it for as long as necessary, until the point is right for the client to look at it themselves.

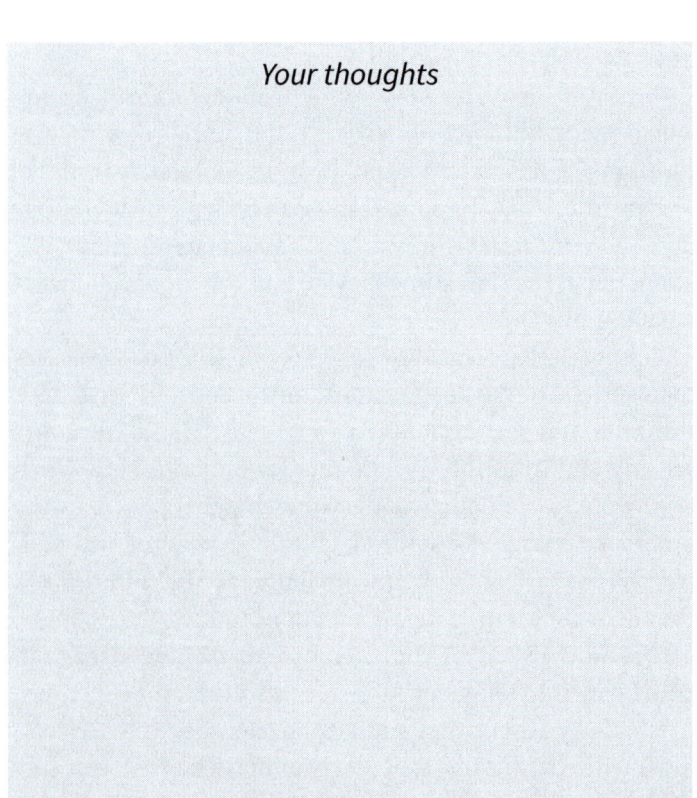

Your thoughts

33

Enriching practice

There are many ways of enhancing the practice of being a therapist. You can enrol for yet another course, one which will introduce a new method, or inform you about how to work with certain special issues. But there seems to me to be a danger that if we immerse ourselves more and more in our professional discipline, we become inward-looking, less in touch with the ordinary world of our clients, and what interests and engages them.

Suppose, for example, instead of asking what CPD you have done this year, you are asked what novels you have read, what films or plays you have seen, how much time you have spent immersed in and observing the natural world. There was a time when one of the professional organisations I belonged to, in its annual review about my CPD over the last year, allowed other ways of learning, which could include studying outside the discipline, or different types of activity. I doubt very much that would be included today. Nevertheless, in reviewing our past year's practice it is worth asking, 'What else have I done? And how has that informed my understanding of people, and the way I work?'

When I read a book, particularly if it's nothing to do with therapy, I find myself triggered into thinking how a character, a particular event, an idea, might inform me about the way some people tick. Often the thought is a passing one, but at other times I feel as if I have learned or understood something really important.

The world of therapy is a fascinating one. It can get hold of you, like a religious faith or a political mission. It can colour the way you think, and indeed it can channel you into thinking about people in a rather narrow way, only meeting in depth people whose lives are often equally narrowed by their particular circumstances.

Before the advent of modern communications, some people would keep a commonplace book, jotting down phrases they had heard, notes about people they had met, situations they had encountered, thoughts that they had had, from their reading, their social life, and their other activities. What a good idea! If you had a commonplace book, in which you could record some of the commonplace things that struck you from books, films, walks, social situations (anything but therapy!) I wonder what they might be? We are amateurs in so many other fields, open to learning about people from different perspectives. There is so much to gain from other disciplines which has bearing upon our work. And daily life has much to teach us as well.

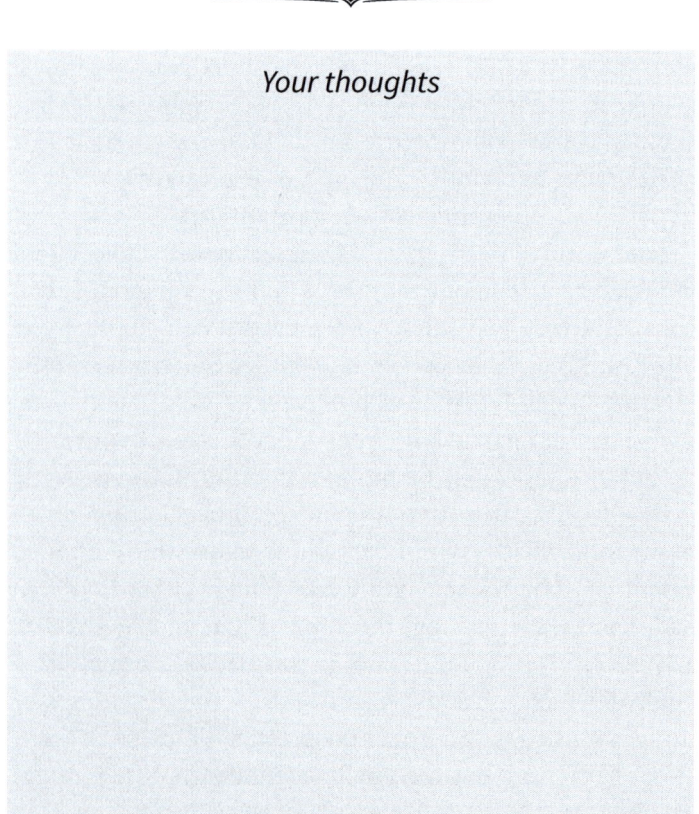

Your thoughts

34

I don't like …

How do you work with someone you don't like? Or with an aspect of them you don't like? The question was raised by Sirote's paper on how the interpersonal therapeutic relationship may stretch the boundaries of usual practice. He describes working with an unpleasant, sinister person, gross in his manner and appearance, who in the course of one session (after he had arrived twenty minutes late), turned to Sirote and said: 'You know, I get the feeling that you just don't like me. Am I right?'[19]

Sirote was 'stupified'. He wondered if he should say that there were things about his patient he did like; or that it wasn't him he disliked but some of what he said or did.

---

[19] Sirote, A. (2015). The patient who had me committed: A mutually influential relationship between patient and analyst in the context of a broadening analytic frame. *Psychoanalytic Perspectives*, *12*: 1–14.

After a long pause thinking about how to respond, he replied, 'To be honest, Raphael, I really don't.'

I don't suggest that this is an example to follow without very careful consideration. In fact, this was some years into a long-term analysis. 'Raphael' had seen other therapists before, so was in one sense a seasoned patient. Nevertheless 'Raphael' was shocked. But this interaction was the turning point in the therapy. Sirote went on to ask, given what they both felt, how they might work together in therapy.

Other therapists have reported how such honesty has been disastrous for the relationship. Sometimes a therapist has pointed out one aspect of the client that the therapist does not like. There is Winnicott's example of the patient who 'was almost loathsome to me for some years'.[20] Winnicott realised, when the therapy had turned a corner, that the patient's 'unlikeableness' was an active symptom, and told the patient that he and the man's friends had once felt repelled by him, but the man had been too ill for Winnicott to let him know.

There will inevitably be features, certain aspects of some of those we work with, that we do not like, or even feel repelled by. Which of these aspects might we bring up in the session? Or do we approach them through generalisations, such as 'I wonder whether you are trying to keep

---

[20] Winnicott, D. W. (1975). Hate in the countertransference. *Through Paediatrics to Psychoanalysis*. London: Hogarth, p. 196.

people (and me?) at a distance?' Would we be able to tell a client about an off-putting manner, or about their body odour? How might we address racist and sexist language which turns us against the client? From irritating dislikes through to full-blown disgust or hatred of the occasional client, we are asked to face our own prejudices, and our cowardice. The reality is that these traits in the client often actually hamper and even prevent the possibility of a healing relationship.

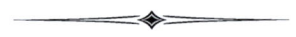

Your thoughts

35

Pressure

When is it right to apply a little pressure upon clients? You may think never at all, since we are (whatever our orientation) in favour of client-led therapy. But you can think of some instances where it is necessary. A client who has not paid you (or your agency), a client who turns up late or misses sessions regularly, and where attempts to understand this pattern get nowhere.

However, in the normal course of things is it helpful to push somewhat in order to, for example, release suppressed feelings, or to confront a defence, to use a rather worn psychodynamic phrase?

Freud asked his patients to speak without censoring their words, as if they were in a railway carriage giving a commentary upon what they saw passing before their eyes. That must have exerted its own pressure. He listened to every detail and every nuance, to every slip of the tongue and every symbol, and shared his understanding of it all.

But did he pressure his patients with his interpretations, as the novelist D. M. Thomas observes, 'when he compels Elizabeth von R. to confront the hidden knowledge that she had been in love with her brother-in-law'?[21] We also know that while he had a forceful personality, he came across to his patients as a kind and caring person, so was it a question of the velvet glove concealing the iron fist?

Pressure can be very subtle, not always obvious. Given that in their training therapists are themselves subjected to strong pressures to conform to the ideas and practices of their teachers and supervisors, it is scarcely surprising that these pressures are internalised and perpetuated in the work with the client—especially if ongoing supervision has a strong teaching element to it. There is pressure to convince the client, as a way of convincing ourselves, that what we have read, what we have been taught, and what we believe must be right. We need a rather special ability to be able to suspend belief in what we have been taught or have even thought through for ourselves, and follow a different path, suggested by the client.

There is, of course, the pressure of time, particularly in situations where either an agency's policy, or the client's limited resources, dictate a set number of sessions, or where the minutes left in a session are limited. Here, time

---

[21] Thomas, D. M. (1982, 13 May). A fine romance. *The New York Review of Books*. https://www.nybooks.com/articles/1982/05/13/a-fine-romance

pressures dictate to the therapist what can and cannot be achieved, and how time can best be managed, but always with the client, and for the benefit of the client.

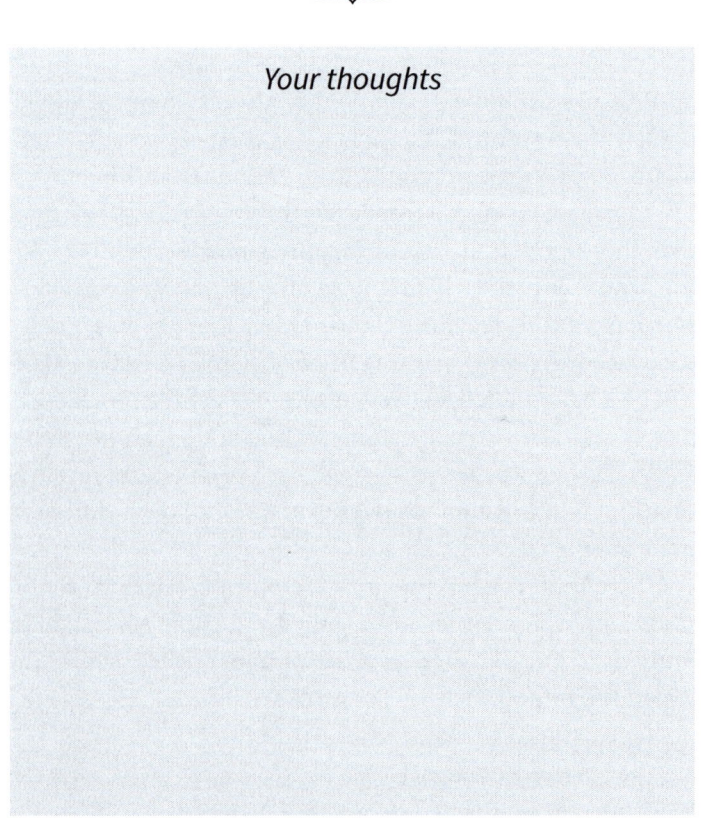

Your thoughts

36

Questions

Michael Balint, who in the mid-twentieth century developed groups for GP's to discuss psychodynamic understanding of their inevitably short consultations with patients,[22] apparently used to say: 'Ask a question, and you'll get an answer. But it won't tell you much!'[23] Nina Coltart quotes this in the context of thinking about silent clients. Although she says that sometimes it is helpful to ask direct questions, she thinks these pressurise the client. Instead she recommends seeking to reassure the client that she is really interested in what they have to say.

She writes in the context of the silent client, but the point is well made for all other work, since asking

---

[22] Balint, M. (1957). *The Doctor, His Patient and the Illness*. London: Churchill Livingstone.

[23] Recounted by Coltart, N. (1991). The silent patient. *Psychoanalytic Dialogues*, 1: 439–453, p. 447.

questions constitutes a type of pressure on the client, who feels obliged to provide an answer so that they do not look foolish or unresponsive. That is one of the reasons why in their training therapists are recommended to ask open questions, which encourage the client to answer in the way they want, which may take the therapy in the direction that is uppermost in the client's mind.

Even open-ended questions suggest that an answer is expected. Questions of any sort may be right for the detective, the chat show host, and the journalist, although their questions are often very closed, and they sometimes ask the obvious. The therapist's questions can sometimes result from the therapist feeling the need to say something (not just with the silent client, but also with the garrulous client), and therefore can interrupt the client's train of thought. Questions may be felt as critical, or as a command, or as a suggestion, none of which, up to that point, had been in the client's mind. As one analyst observed, 'each patient brings a unique prior life experience concerning asking and being asked questions'.[24]

Questions may be necessary at times, yet I wonder, if we looked closely at conversations that take place in close relationships, between friends or partners, whether they would

---

[24] Boesky, D. (1990). The questions and curiosity of the psychoanalyst. *Journal of the American Psychoanalytic Association*, *37*: 579–603, p. 602.

feature very much, except perhaps as rhetorical questions (such as this one)? In other words, isn't the rhetorical type of question not only about what interests me, but also what I think might interest you? Therefore it invites a dialogue, rather than suggesting that there is a piece of information which I need and which you can supply—which will make me feel better, but may not be at this point in time relevant to you.

Dare I ask, 'What do you think?'

Your thoughts

37

Difference

'It was from the difference between us, not from the affinities and likenesses but from the difference, that that love came'. The love the narrator refers to is the relationship between two complete strangers, who in their sexuality and gender are completely different, one a male from earth but on a foreign planet, the other an androgyne, who can be either 'male' or 'female' in procreation. Their cultures are therefore completely different too.[25]

In an introduction to *The Left Hand of Darkness*, David Mitchell comments that 'there is no difficulty or achievement in understanding someone who is already very like you'.[26] We therapists talk a lot about empathy, but is empathy really possible when relating to someone who in some respects is completely different from yourself? I suggest

---

[25] Le Guin, U. (1969). *The Left Hand of Darkness*. London: Futura.
[26] Kindle version of *The Left Hand of Darkness*, location 103.

not, at least not without that person first telling you about their own experience of being who they are. We simply cannot imagine it. Nor can we be certain, if we meet the same difference again but with someone else, that we can understand them through empathy. Empathy requires of us the ability to put ourselves in the position of the other, so as to try to imagine what it must be like to be them. I am not sure that this is ever straightforward, even if that person is 'already very like you'.

In matters of sexuality and gender there are some deep divisions in our own culture, and even deeper in some other cultures on our own and other continents. We may think, because our training has emphasised empathy, that if we get into the other's frame of mind, we can speak to that person sensitively, and grasp what it feels like to be them, even when who they are and their circumstances are alien to us.

But there is another side to this which is implicit in the novel's portrayal of the relationship between two people who are in some or many respects different. For there to be a deep relationship, each person has firstly to want the other to speak their truth; and secondly to want their relationship to be able to absorb their deep differences. It raises the question of whether we can comprehend the other just by empathising with them. It is not just that we want the other to speak about themselves without fear of our criticism or prejudice. A deep relationship also requires that the other can understand us and the ways we are similar and different from them. Perhaps the closest relationships are such, not just because we each understand what we have in common, but because we each recognise and accept difference.

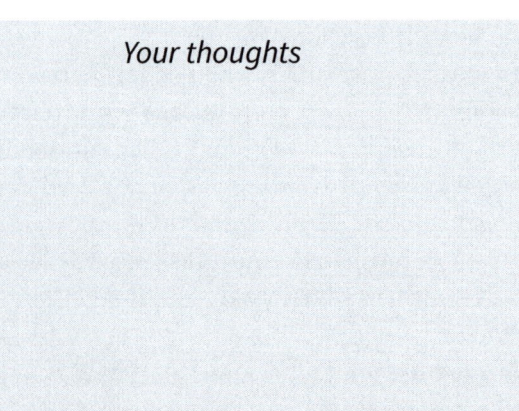

Your thoughts

38

Remembering

There's one feature of memory which fascinates me. It is what I can only call a tit-bit, something we heard from the client long ago, that suddenly pops into my mind in the middle of a session, as if from nowhere. It may not be a tit-bit after all, since it is as if our unconscious is telling us something about the person we are listening to, which connects with what they are saying now. It can be of real significance.

Another aspect of remembering is when we find ourselves thinking about someone we have seen in therapy, perhaps many years ago. We can remember them as much when we are outside the therapy room as when we are in it, when we are getting on with something else. Many of us remember very well the first client we ever saw, although we may not necessarily remember a huge amount about them—rather the way we got on, and what we felt for each other. But it can happen with any client, even someone we only met for a single session. We may be reminded of what they looked like, perhaps how good it was working with them, perhaps, on the other hand, recalling, at that point, a difficult session; something we may have said which we got wrong; or perhaps something we said which proved a turning point.

I do not know what it means, except that where we once held people in mind in the sessions with them, the way they pop into our head, seems to show that we still hold them in mind. We have not the slightest idea in the majority of instances of where they are, whether they are alive or dead, what they went on to achieve or whether nothing ever changed for them, how much they had ever gained from their relationship with us, or not. Occasionally we may of course hear from one of them: perhaps a card at Christmas, maybe even a letter catching us up on where they are now, or even a request for further help. But the vast majority we never see or hear from again. Nevertheless they are still there, held in mind.

These rememberings seem important, although I don't know why. We reconnect with people who have mattered to us in the past, and we think well of them—easy with most; and easier at this distance if we did not think quite so well of them at the time. And in all probability they remember us, perhaps more often than we remember them, but in the same way as we remember our own therapist. That's rather nice.

Your thoughts

39

What did you miss out?

Following the live broadcast of an episode of 'In Our Time' on BBC Radio 4, the host Melvyn Bragg asks his guests, who have been talking with him about a specific subject for forty-five minutes: 'What did you miss out, that you would like to have said?' In the podcast of the programme, off air, that discussion is broadcast with the main programme.

Melvyn probably wants to give his guests the opportunity to add something which his guidance of the topic on air gave insufficient space for them to contribute. He may also have in mind that talking together, possibly more relaxed when not on air, may trigger aspects of the subject which did not occur to them during the main broadcast.

Following a therapy session therapists usually write notes, which include summaries of what the client said, and/or what the therapist said, the therapist's experience and the observed client experience of the session, as well as, on occasion, ideas that occur to the therapist afterwards, which did not occur to the therapist at the time, but might be useful to bear in mind for future sessions. I wonder whether there might be another aspect to the record a therapist makes, that can be thought about then or later, perhaps in supervision: 'What did I think of saying that I didn't say and why didn't I say it?'

What is interesting here is the second part of that question: 'Why did I not say it?' There are going to be different reasons, which are themselves worth reflecting upon. Perhaps I didn't say it because the client was in full flow and I did not want to interrupt; and by the time the client had paused it did not seem relevant. Perhaps I did not say it because I hadn't processed it enough to be sure it would be helpful. It might be a good idea to pursue the thought and see whether it could be relevant another time. Perhaps the reason was that I was afraid I would upset the client—'upset' meaning either that I would distress the client too much, or that I would make the client angry. Perhaps it was that I was not sure I could take the client's response, protecting myself, whereas it actually would have been the right thing to say. That might mean that I need to look at myself and whether I avoid certain reactions and topics. Perhaps I did not say it because it was my own agenda, and I can be thankful I kept quiet. It would have been irrelevant: or would it possibly still be relevant, and needs some thinking about before I can use it?

Your thoughts

40

His (or her or their) therapist's voice

How are you heard? The psychoanalyst Herbert Rosenfeld makes the point that some patients listen closely to their analyst's voice, and its tone, but that they do not hear what the analyst actually says. He observes that there are some analysts whose voice is so expressionless that it has a deadening effect on the patient.[27] And the problem is that these analysts do not know how damaging an expressionless voice can be.

He makes the point that those who come to therapy, especially at the very beginning, are sensitive to every nuance of the setting—this obviously includes the furnishing and ambience of the room, but it also includes the way the therapist speaks. The client is alert to whether the

---

[27] Rosenfeld, H. (1987). *Impasse and Interpretation: Therapeutic and Anti-therapeutic Factors in the Psychoanalytic Treatment of Psychotic, Borderline and Neurotic Patients.* London: Tavistock, p. 279

therapist sounds critical, impatient, tired, rushed, etc. And this applies throughout the work. The therapist's voice may convey to the client that the therapist feels warm or cold towards them, even if it is not the way the therapist actually feels. The tone may be one of tiredness or liveliness, engagement or distance.

This made me wonder about a distinction that Nina Coltart made between the way she is when working as a psychotherapist and the way she is when she is working as an analyst. Unfortunately what she says bears out the stereotypical picture of the analyst, which is probably not what she wanted to convey. She writes that in psychotherapy 'I would allow freer rein to my spontaneity, and would not be afraid of expressing more emotion, of whatever kind, than I would if engaged on a full analysis'.[28] She includes jokes and laughing as part of some sessions if it felt right.

One reviewer of Coltart's book says that it sounds as if psychotherapy is more engaging for therapist and patient but less committed. It sounds to me as if it is more engaging and more committed. And, like the reviewer, I am not at all sure, although I do not have that experience, that psychoanalysis as distinct from psychotherapy is as buttoned-up as Coltart makes it sound.

---

[28] Coltart, N. (1993). *How to Survive as a Psychotherapist*. London: Sheldon Press, p. 16.

Therapists differ in their manner—some come across in voice and gesture as more serious, others as lighter, some as more fluid in their movements, and some as rather more tranquil. This is not to advocate exaggerated 'emoting' or false jollity, but it is to validate genuine feelings as a therapist when it feels that it would be right to share these with the client. And when you speak, do your voice and manner truly convey your thoughts and feelings to your client?

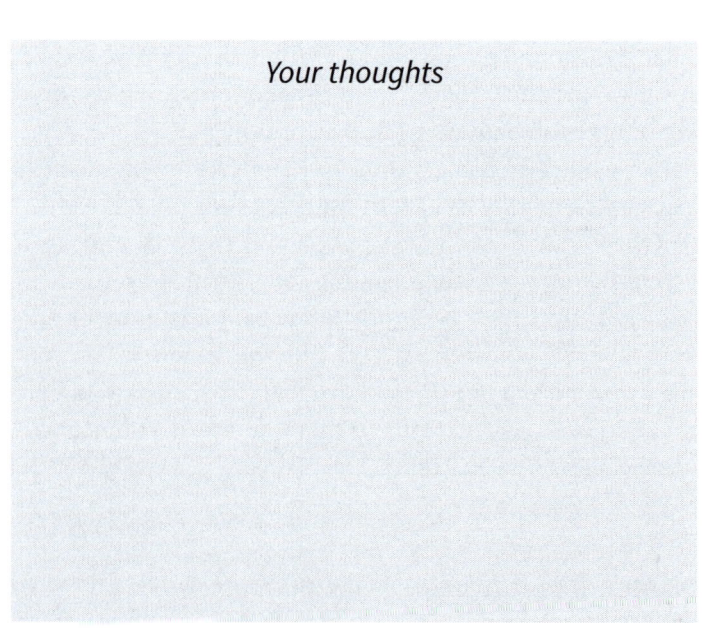

Your thoughts

41

Hope

A number of journal articles about hope in therapy cite a passage where Winnicott quotes one of his patients: 'The only time I felt hope was when you told me that you [i.e. Winnicott] could see no hope, and you continued with the analysis.'[29]

It is difficult to imagine a therapist saying 'I cannot see any hope', and I wonder whether those were the actual words Winnicott (or indeed his patient) actually used. Winnicott explains that this patient had previously been a long time with another analyst who did not seem to have realised that the patient consistently presented a false self. Winnicott implies that he was challenging his patient that if they could work to find his true self, then there could be hope. Perhaps that justified what looks like a rather

---

[29] Winnicott, D. W. (1965). *The Maturational Processes and the Facilitating Environment*. London: Hogarth, p. 152.

damning statement, although there is consolation in Winnicott saying, as it were, 'Nevertheless, we will go on working together, whatever happens'.

Suppose we consider false hope as well as the false self. Hope is a wishful illusion, specifically referring to the future, when what the future holds is unknown, and where there may or may not be evidence to support that hope. Hope provides the incentive to do things, to plan things, to believe that what comes our way will be largely benign, because hope is built on the basis of evidence from past experiences and our present situation. Where a person has had a past which has largely crushed hope, which instead has generated dread, then it follows that the future is coloured by the futility that accompanies hopelessness. Where past hopes have turned out to be false hopes, future hopes stand little chance of ever being realised. No wonder hope turns into despair.

What Winnicott seems to me to be saying is that there is no hope in wishing things will change in the future, since past experience does not give any confidence that it can. A therapist does not know what the future holds, and simply to work on the basis of hope is false therapy. There is no chance of any hope unless therapy can address the crushing of hope in the past, the absence of consolation when it was most needed, and when the evidence so far leads to the conclusion that there is no hope. There can be no hope when the grim reality of the past and the present informs a person's view of the future. Nevertheless, what can be offered, when there is no hope, is a commitment to go on working, come what may. The best hope that can be offered (with a pretty reasonable chance of being fulfilled) is 'We'll meet again next week'.

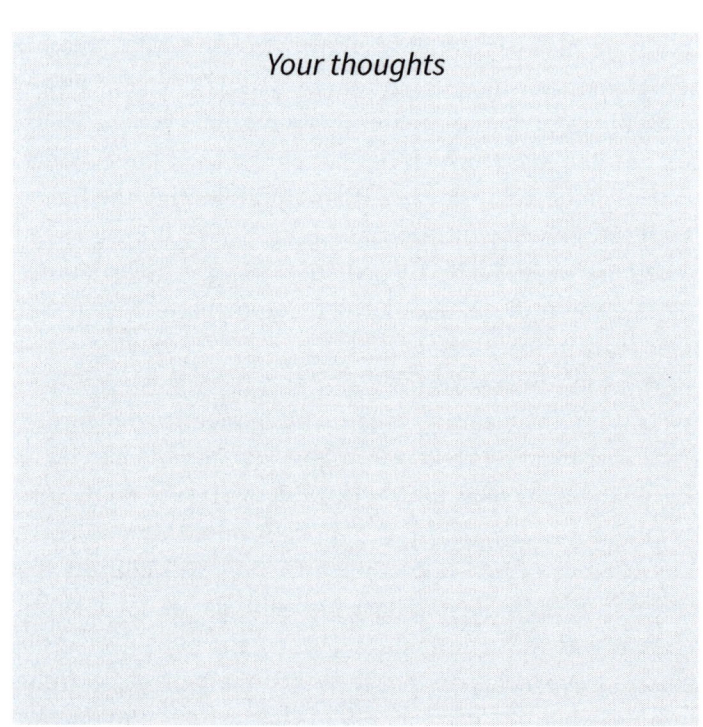

Your thoughts

42

Gifts

One of the best examples of how to work with the offer of presents by clients is Joy Schaverien's account of the various gifts which a patient of hers gave her or tried to give her.[30] The way she handles these situations is a lesson on how to accept gifts; and how, after considering their meaning, to refuse them. Schaverien makes a distinction between a gift as a token and a gift as a talisman, a talisman being a gift which is intended to have a magical effect. For example, a gift of flowers could be a token of friendship or gratitude. Or it could be an attempt to propitiate the therapist, as if the patient thinks the therapist is angry with them. Or it can be a way of reacting against the patient's own anger with the therapist. It can

---

[30] Schaverien, J. (2011). Gifts, talismans and tokens in analysis: Symbolic enactments or sinister acts? *Journal of Analytical Psychology*, 56: 160–183.

be a way of preventing the therapist from forgetting them during a break, or a way of trying to ensure that the therapist will love them whatever happens.

The gift as a talisman has many possible rich meanings in the context of the therapeutic relationship, which ask to be understood. Joy Schaverien concludes her case example with a lovely description of her recognising that her patient wanted to bring a gift as they concluded the therapy; and discussing the possible meaning of the various ideas with the patient about what she might give her. Finally, having worked through the different possibilities, they settled together on the actual gift which the therapist was happy to accept.

There are other types of gift which need to be considered in relation to this question of how best to work with them. A client may bring a poem or a picture which they want to share or give to the therapist, which clearly can be full of meaning. I do not forget what a therapist gives: their attention and their experience, a deep sense of wanting to do as much as is possible for the client; and offers toleration and acceptance to the client who is not easy to like, or whom the therapist might in other circumstances not want to share time with.

There is a sense in which everything which a client brings to the session is a gift, something they want to share with the therapist, and something they want to leave with the therapist, to be given back, enriched later in therapy, as in Edward Thomas' poem 'And You, Helen': 'If I could choose / Freely in that great treasure-house / Anything from any shelf / I would give you back yourself'.[31]

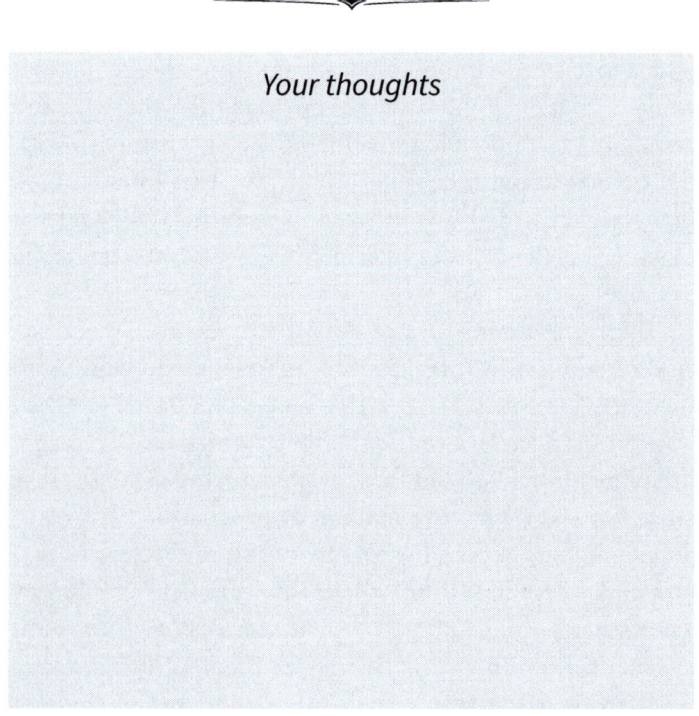

Your thoughts

[31] Thomas, R. G. (1978). *The Poems of Edward Thomas*. Oxford: Oxford University Press.

43

Leaving therapy

I wondered why I had never thought of doing it: I was looking at recent psychoanalytic thinking about endings.[32] For a start it seemed, thank goodness, that the phrase 'termination of therapy' is gradually being dropped. It smacks too much of death, abortion, and finality, as though (indeed this was once the thinking) when therapy ends it is for good, when everything that could be achieved has been achieved and 'the transference' dissolved. It is obvious too that instead of the notion that it is the analyst who decides when it is best to end, ending is a process, which involves both therapist and client, each of whom has obvious feelings about it, as well as ideas as to when it will be most appropriate. These days, of course, much therapy on the NHS and in counselling centres has to be limited,

---

[32] Frank, K. A. (2009). Ending with options. *Psychoanalytic Inquiry*, *29*: 136–156.

and an end date is either set (or preferably negotiated) at the very start. The ending is a feature of dynamic short-term work from the very start. But would it be right also in open-ended therapy to talk in the beginning about how the ending will be managed when the time comes for therapy to finish?

Another aspect that I had never considered as built in to the process of ending is the offer of a review session six months after the final session (or perhaps in the case of time-limited short-term work, six weeks on). The finality of ending—termination—has been challenged, with some therapists now clearly offering a follow-up session to the client. Obviously, this again is discussed with the client, who may or may not want to accept the offer, and a date can be set at the time. This is arranged as a review, not starting therapy again, although this may be considered at that time for the particularly vulnerable if it is practical for both parties.

I then thought of medical practice, where consultants often build a review into their work with a patient, after a year, and even sometimes for several years running. Given the more personal and intense relationship in psychotherapy, why do we therapists not do the same? I had always been open to a client returning for further therapy, but I had never considered building in a review as part of the ending process.

Given the nature of the therapeutic relationship, is it right to finish just like that—however much the ending has been negotiated and worked through? If a friend is moving away so that we will not see them so regularly, it would be surprising if we never met again. The therapy relationship is often as close as, or in some ways closer than, friendship. Surely it cannot be dismissed just like that?

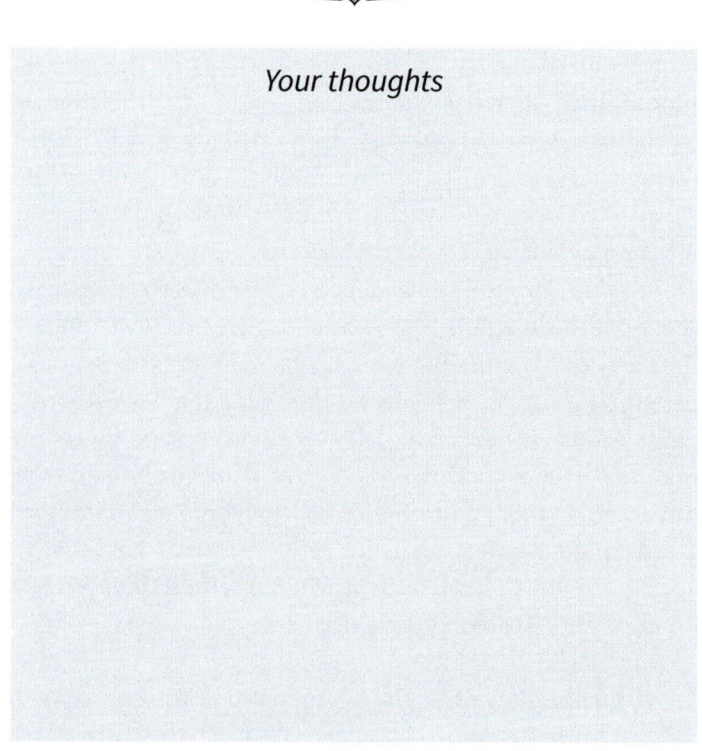

Your thoughts

44

Alone or lonely?

The distinction between aloneness and loneliness is well recognised: we can be lonely in a crowd, and we can be content, even glad, to be alone. This 'capacity to be alone', Winnicott's phrase,[33] develops from the ability as a child to be alone and to play alone in the presence of a silent yet protective other, leading to the ability to be alone with ourselves, whatever our various selves are experiencing.

I think here of the loneliness and the aloneness of being a therapist, although it must apply to a large number of professional and leisure activities. Alone with a book, alone in the countryside, or in a busy town; the writer, the student, the artist and the craftsperson. We can feel especially lonely when what we are wanting to achieve does not work,

---

[33] Winnicott, D. W. (1965). *The Maturational Processes and the Facilitating Environment*. London: Hogarth, pp. 29–36.

cannot be grasped, cannot be understood, and leaves us feeling dissatisfied, especially if we have invested much. When we can share that feeling and what has led to it with another, it may help. Loneliness converts into aloneness when the therapist can draw upon the theories and practices which their training has promoted and supported.

Therapy can be immensely rewarding; but it can also undermine our confidence when what we try to do doesn't work; when what we wanted to achieve is precious to us, and failure leaves us feeling bereft. Loneliness as a therapist is liable to occur, and stay with us, when what we have learned proves worthless. We have very little to fall back on. A client, in one way or another, chews up what we offer, or refuses to engage in working together, or spills it all out but is in no mood to hear what we have to say. We are on our own without the support of all we have learned. Helplessness breeds loneliness. And although these experiences can be shared with another, no amount of wise supervisory suggestions take away that feeling of working with such a client.

There is just the possibility that our loneliness reflects the client's sense of uselessness and loneliness. We can perhaps speak of the experience that the two of us are probably going through, simultaneously but individually; and awaken, again perhaps, the client's awareness that their experience is not unique. Loneliness converts into aloneness in the session when both therapist and client fall into a contented or meditative silence where each supports the other's wish to be alone and silent for the time being. That we have shared together in a therapeutic moment enables us to enjoy being alone. When therapist and patient can be alone in the presence of the other, it is a remarkable achievement.

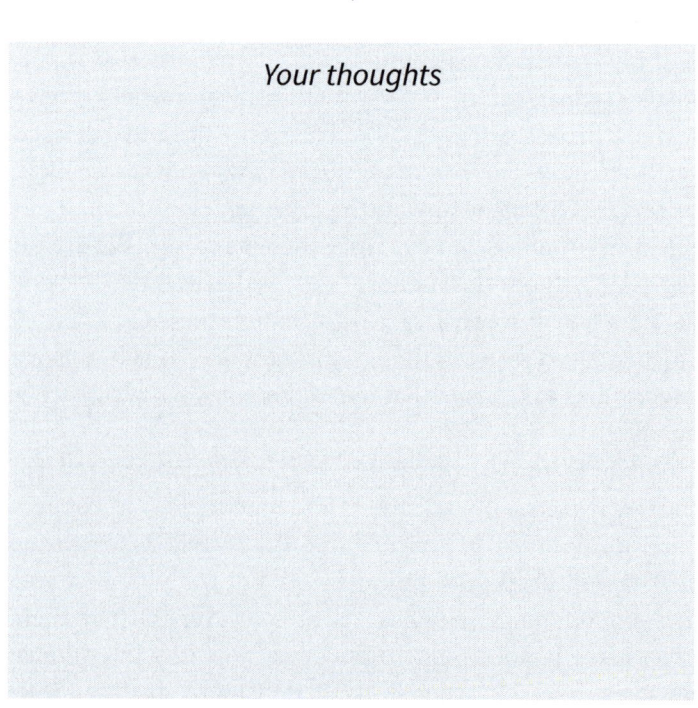

Your thoughts

45

Taboo

It used to be said of conversations in polite society, particularly round the dinner table, that the three subjects to be avoided were sex, death, and religion. That may still apply not just to the dinner table, but also to many relationships, including to those who are in committed partnerships.

Sex and death are of course the two main drives that Freud identified as being at the root of psychological distress. Love and aggression might be a more nuanced way of putting it, but for the moment let us consider these raw desires and fears, and how much they feature in therapeutic conversations. There are some presentations which concern either or both of those issues.

Sexual problems can be the reason people seek therapy, although those who have relationship issues do not necessarily talk intimately about their sexual life, their fantasies and the realities. Is it possible that sex is still a taboo subject when it comes to oneself even if, as far as society and the media are concerned, there appears on the surface to be no issue? Is it all out there, in the media, but not actually something people talk about when it comes to themselves?

And those who have been bereaved naturally talk about the death of those they have lost. There is much richness in working with bereavement, although we cannot skate over grief when it involves a death many years ago. Nearly everyone has experienced deaths which they have never really had the chance to fully grieve, particularly those that occurred in childhood and young adulthood. Do we also talk about our own death? For the young it probably seems a long way off, and therefore not as relevant as it is later in life. That is possibly another taboo subject even though it is an inevitable part of ageing.

Taboos vary and may not be universal. It is clearly important that therapists try to discover what the taboo areas might be in a particular person's upbringing. Even if these need to be as much part of the therapy conversation as anything else, sensitivity to taboos is equally necessary. We have to think of how we introduce forbidden areas into the conversation, how we make them safe to be discussed, and how we distinguish thinking and speaking about taboo areas from doing and acting. Likewise, just because we and our clients have not acted out taboos, it doesn't mean that we and they haven't thought about them and felt them.

Most important of all, we as therapists have to face our own taboos. Perhaps there are certain subjects, certain emotions, certain fantasies, which we prefer not to think about and certainly feel anxious raising with clients. Then there are specific taboos for therapy itself. It is worth wondering how much the strength of those taboos inhibit us in what we think and say.

Your thoughts

46

Money

Therapists and counsellors, unless they are very fortunate, have to earn a living. That means charging for their services. That involves a heavy outlay for some clients and makes therapy impossible to access for many people. Yet we must charge a fee.

A survey of sixty therapists found that two-thirds of them experienced inner conflict about setting fees. Women therapists were rather more conflicted than men, and those from families where money has been an issue appear to have more conflict than others.[34] One source suggests there are different attitudes to fee-setting: some discuss fees with the client, enquire into their finances and tailor the fee accordingly. Others set high fees to satisfy their sense of professional worth. Some do not discuss the fee at all and

[34] Lasky. E. (1984). Psychoanalysts' and psychotherapists' conflicts about setting fees. *Psychoanalytic Psychology*, *1*: 289–300.

give the client no opportunity to agree it. Others ask too little or leave the fee to the client.[35]

In setting fees, the place to start is how many sessions a therapist can reasonably offer, and how much work can they undertake without becoming emotionally exhausted and over-tired. Self-care is high on the list of ethical requirements in most professional associations. The second question is how many sessions are likely to be active at any one time. Then the therapist can set this figure against how much they need to earn, bearing in mind what other income they may have, or may need to source in order to keep their fee at a reasonable level.

However, a therapist may wish to offer a lower fee to potential clients who could not otherwise afford it. Similarly, if sessions are missed with or without warning, how much of the fee should be required, if at all? These considerations and estimates may mean that those who can afford therapy have to pay more to enable those who cannot afford the full fee to have therapy; or pay more to allow for missed sessions.

There is also the question of raising the fee as the cost-of-living increases for therapist and client alike. Where fees are variable, how might you react with a client changing

---

[35] Riemann, F. (1968). The personality structure of the analyst and its influence on the course of treatment. *The American Journal of Psychoanalysis*, *28*: 69–79.

jobs, or coming into money and significantly increasing their income? Or their income decreasing: suppose, for example, a client decides to train for another career, a move which is an indication of their psychological progress?

All these variables need to be considered when working out fee structures. Having worked through these questions, therapists will be in a better position to work with conflicts about money that arise with clients.

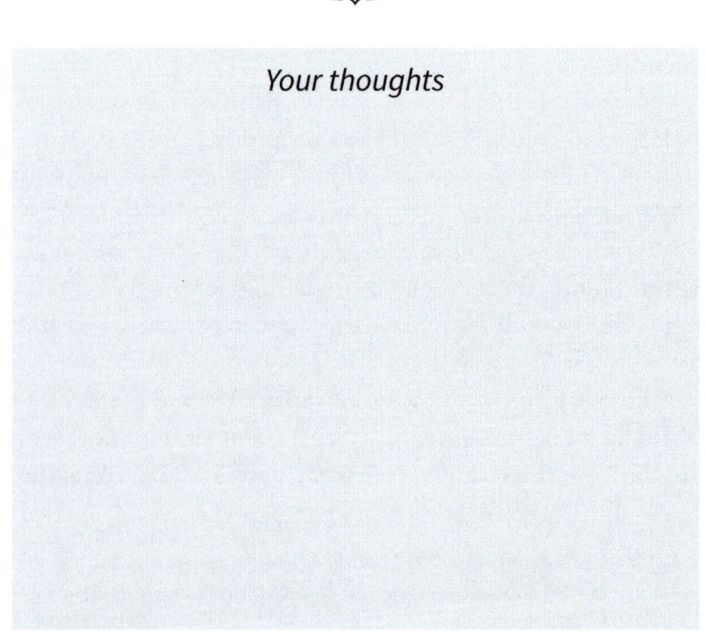

Your thoughts

47

Does one size really fit all?

There is considerable emphasis in a psychodynamic training on the frame—which includes the time, the timing, and frequency of sessions—usually once weekly (in the case of counselling, and in practice for most psychotherapy), at the same time, and for fifty minutes. There is a sense in which the frame is inviolable, so that any infringement of the boundaries needs to be addressed and understood. I do not disagree, but I am also concerned about therapy becoming entrenched in hard and fast rules, into which clients must fit.

As several therapists argue, the frame is both a structure and a process.[36] We have to have a structure for our work, and we seem to expect clients to fit the structure, without really involving them in the process of creating

---

[36] For example, Gabbard, G. (2007). Flexibility of the frame re-visited. *Psychoanalytic Dialogues*, *17*(6): 923–929.

a structure with them. Do sessions have to last fifty minutes for everyone? There are some clients who would find a shorter session less threatening—I remember a client asking for two twenty-minute sessions a week rather than one fifty-minute session. It worked well in helping him cope with the stress of his disturbed inner world; as well as by him taking the initiative for what he needed for himself. Others may not get into their stride easily given the limit of fifty minutes and need longer. What if forty-five minutes became the usual length, to allow the therapist more time to reflect afterwards on sessions? The best length of a session may not become clear until after several sessions. That could be the point for negotiation of the optimum time for each individual. Then the frame is constructed between the two parties, and it is that which becomes generally inviolable.

There is also the question of how to manage a session which atypically needs to go on longer. This can be negotiated with the client, rather than either letting it happen or ignoring the possibility of a short extension. 'Would a few extra minutes help?', we may ask, when it is clear that calling time is at a point when the client is likely to leave the room either carrying some distress, or not having fully expressed the feelings that have been brought to the fore.

The difference between this approach and a totally informal, unstructured, potentially chaotic, disturbing and uncontained arrangement, is that our work engages clients in the process from the very beginning. After all, we want them, when we finally finish the therapy, to take the best of what we have done together. Tailor-made—not off the shelf.

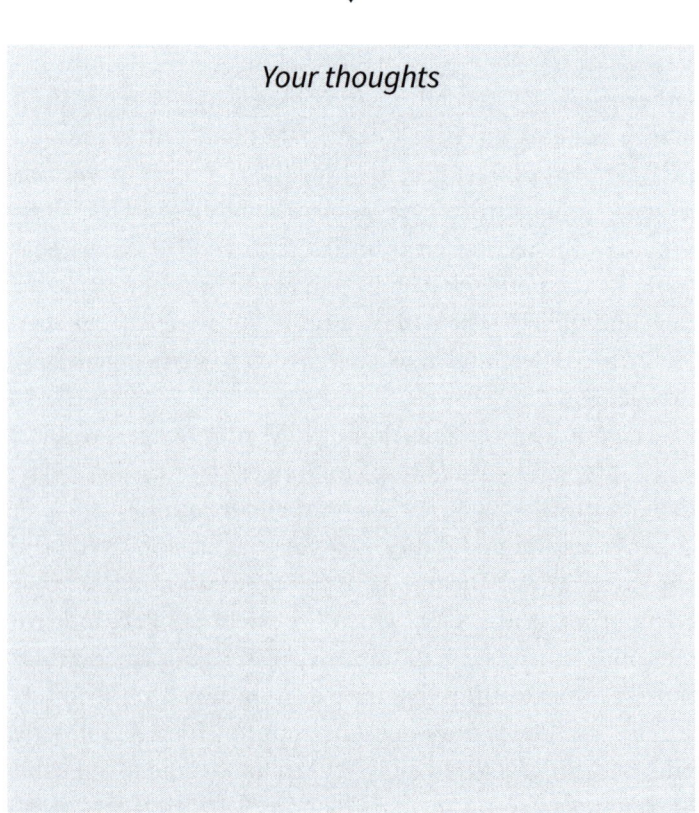

Your thoughts

48

Notes

How astonishing—a performance of Mozart's 'Jupiter' symphony where the whole orchestra plays from memory: or another orchestra plays Stravinsky's *Rite of Spring*—again completely from memory. But then don't all of us remember tunes and whistle or sing along to music of all kinds, better perhaps than we remember the words of poems that we have also heard several times?

Our memories are astonishing. As we listen to clients, we find ourselves remembering events, places, and people that they have told us about, sometimes only once and many weeks ago. It is clear too that the more we are engaged with a client, and the more we are moved and interested in what they are telling us, the more they strike a chord and the more we remember.

Which makes me wonder why we make notes to remind us of the content of sessions, when it may only be necessary to write down anything more of what was said than some of the basic facts—names, dates, places. We will surely remember what happened, what the client felt, and the effect on the client as long as we give them proper attention. After all, we do not record the conversations we have with friends and yet we remember much about what we have talked about with them.

Might there be a better way of using the time between sessions, or at the end of the day, to reflect instead of recording what happened and what was said. I have suggested elsewhere in these pages that we might want to record what we did not say but wished we had said. We might also record what we did not say but could not say. We might, since notes are a way of improving our practice, ask ourselves what we have learned in the session that we had not realised before.

I do not question the value of verbatim notes in training, for some supervision, and when we are initially learning our craft. Neither do I question the necessity of recording the details when we are told about experiences of abuse, which may at some time even in the distant future be needed for legal purposes. But I do suggest that there may be more fruitful ways of reflecting on the session, pointing to future sessions rather than what has just passed. If we trust our unconscious and allow it to release memories into consciousness when needed, then our memories of what has transpired in past sessions will be triggered when relevant in the here and now.

Recording notes can easily become a paper exercise. How might you design your record sheet so that it becomes more reflective, and more creative?

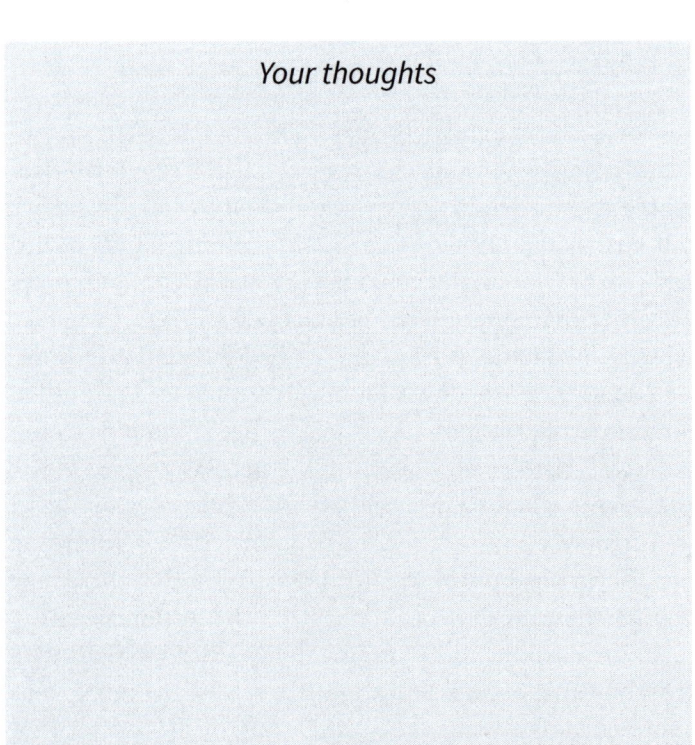

Your thoughts

49

Co-creation

As the reader will be aware, I draw considerably upon the creative ideas that appear in the writing of psychoanalysts, some well-known, others to me only a name at the top of a journal article. Although I do not know them personally, they help me develop my own thinking and practice. Their creativity inspires my own. Yet in my writing it has always been the clients who have fine-tuned or even made me rethink my ideas. Therapy is essentially a creative process, with therapist and client co-creators. That does not mean that therapy always produces positive outcomes. Therapy can create chaos as well, and again that chaos comes from the interaction of therapist and client, not only from one side, whether it be the ineptitude of the therapist or the disasters of the client's experience.

While I enjoy the stimulus of psychoanalytic ideas, I am not so keen on labelling therapy as analytic—as in psychoanalytic, analytical psychology, or transactional analysis. The term smacks too much of the medical or the scientific model, trying to discover or uncover what has gone wrong, as though we are static creatures, who have had experiences that are carved in stone, waiting to be cleaned up and interpreted. What we hear in therapy are the ways in which a client perceives their experiences at this point in time, with this particular therapist.

Clients paint word pictures for us, they create their stories as they recreate their experience, as they show us their feelings and they reveal their thoughts. This is no mere uncovering, nor is our task merely discovering; we are together engaged in a creative process, at the micro as well as at the macro level of therapy. As I respond to a client's story, I add suggestions of my own to the script, and the client in turn refines what I have said.

As David Mark writes: 'More and more, analysts of all persuasions regard interpretations as creating something … rather than simply discovering something hidden inside the patient'.[37] Likewise he suggests that empathy is not discovering a person's experience, but is a particular way of listening whereby the fallible therapist tries to get hold of the client's experience. It is, therefore, a creation of the imagination.

---

[37] Mark, D. (2006). 'I never knew I was a democrat': Discovery and creation in psychoanalysis. *Contemporary Psychoanalysis*, *42*: 85–105, p. 86.

The way clients choose, consciously and unconsciously, to tell their stories, similarly demonstrates their creativity, in what they choose to include and what they leave out, in the words they use, in the expression they give to those words, in the feelings they evoke in themselves and in us. The therapist is not the interpreter of those stories, but, at first, the listener, and then, the co-creator, as the therapist adds to the narrative, selecting some aspects, putting aside others, developing from their own creative spirit.

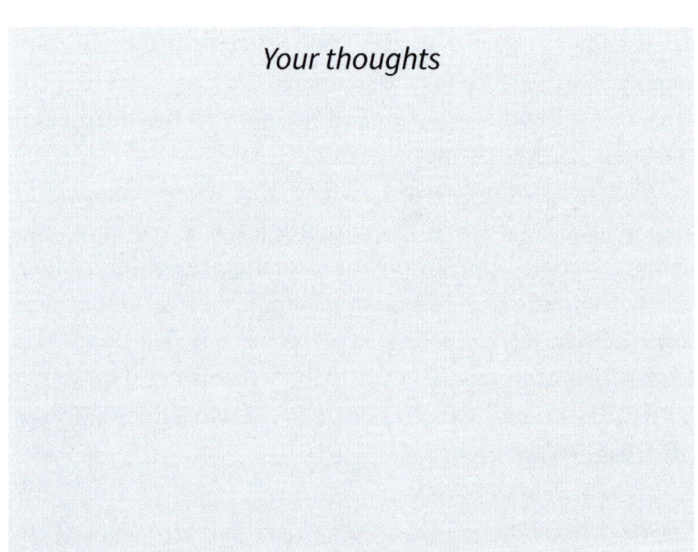

Your thoughts

50

The mysterium

Freud called religion an illusion and denied that he had ever experienced the oceanic feelings to which his correspondent, the poet Romain Rolland, referred. He set the tone in early psychoanalysis for a view of spirituality, as well as of religion, that claimed it was an escape, a defence, a false solution to issues that engender fear—such as death. It was left to Jung and his followers to fly the flag for the spiritual. It is noticeable, however, that in contemporary psychoanalysis the interest in spiritual experience has reappeared, from a more sympathetic and positive stance.

I have problems with using the term 'spiritual' because it can be interpreted in so many ways. It can mean religious belief and practices; it can mean meditation or mindfulness; it can mean being moved by music, poetry, art, etc. All these forms have the ability to open us to enriching experiences, and in turn to psychological and intellectual satisfaction. Therapists need to be open to a client's religious or spiritual references, and to looking with them at both the enhancing and inhibiting aspects of their unique spirituality.

What I have in mind as I reflect, however, is something other: that is, awareness in therapists of the place of the numinous, of the unknown, of the mysterium, of (and this is where Freud showed his interest) the uncanny. Therapists, as is frequently cited in the literature, need to be (in Keats' words) 'capable of being in uncertainties, mysteries, doubts, without any irritable reaching after fact or reason'. There is much which as individuals we do not know or understand, although in many instances there are others who apparently do: some of our unknowns others know and in theory could explain to us. But this is only a small part of the unknown I have in mind. There is much that is unknown that waits to be discovered, or in therapy to be experienced, which is why therapy is part of a lifelong process. Even that is still a small part of the unknown that I have in mind. What I really have in mind, but find very difficult, if not impossible to describe (although you may yourself also have had glimpses of its significance), is the ultimate unknown, a glimpsed perception of the otherness which is not us, yet of which we are also a part.

I have in mind something larger than psychotherapy and counselling, something much greater than the physical and the philosophical, something which evokes a sense of amazement at its unknownness, a sense of awe yet without accompanying fear and anxiety, a sense of reverence yet without having to invent a god or a religion, a sense of fascination without the need to explain or define or to ask further questions. Such unknownness endows us with humility as we engage with clients, colleagues, friends, and family, with this otherwise all-consuming life and with our inner world.

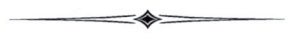

Your thoughts

About the author

Michael Jacobs is one of the pioneers of psychodynamic counselling and therapy in Britain. Of his many books, he is best known for *Psychodynamic Counselling in Action* and *The Presenting Past*. Thinking back on over fifty years' experience as a therapist and supervisor, Michael invites the reader to pause and reflect with him on some of the fascinating and crucial aspects of the therapeutic relationship.